# Immunity

## How to Use Yoga for Improved Health and Wellness

*(Proven Strategies to Improve Your Immune System During Pandemic)*

## Edward Sanchez

Published By **Jordan Levy**

# Edward Sanchez

All Rights Reserved

*Immunity: How to Use Yoga for Improved Health and Wellness (Proven Strategies to Improve Your Immune System During Pandemic)*

**ISBN   978-1-7752619-9-5**

Legal & Disclaimer

The information contained in this book is not designed to replace or take the place of any form of medicine or professional medical advice. The information in this book has been provided for educational & entertainment purposes only.

The information contained in this book has been compiled from sources deemed reliable, and it is accurate to the best of the Author's knowledge; however, the Author cannot guarantee its accuracy and validity and cannot be held liable for any errors or omissions. Changes are periodically made to this book. You must consult your doctor or get professional medical advice before using any of the suggested remedies, techniques, or information in this book.

Table Of Contents

## Chapter 1: Building A Strong Foundation

The Mind-Body Connection

The thoughts-frame connection is a complex and complicated dating between our highbrow and bodily fitness. It refers back to the way in which our mind, feelings, and behaviors could have an effect on our bodily health and vice versa. The thoughts-frame connection has been studied considerably in ultra-modern years, and studies has tested that there may be a sturdy hyperlink among our mental and bodily health. In this article, we will discover the thoughts-body connection and its effect on Psychological Immunity.

Psychological Immunity refers to our capability to address stress, adversity, and demanding situations in existence. It is an critical element of our highbrow fitness and nicely-being. The thoughts-frame connection plays a crucial role in Psychological Immunity, as our intellectual and physical fitness are intently intertwined. When we revel in strain or adversity, our frame responds in numerous strategies, which includes elevated heart rate, muscle tension, and adjustments in respiratory. These bodily responses are part of our frame's natural safety mechanism, designed to assist us cope with pressure and adversity.

However, whilst strain and adversity end up chronic, our frame's safety mechanism can turn out to be overactive, most crucial to quite more than a few bodily and highbrow fitness troubles. Chronic stress has been linked to more than a few health troubles, along with coronary coronary heart disorder, diabetes, and despair. The mind-frame connection plays a important position on this device, as our mind, emotions, and behaviors can exacerbate or alleviate the physical signs and symptoms and symptoms of stress.

For example, people who experience persistent pressure may additionally additionally increase horrible idea styles, which includes catastrophizing or rumination. These horrible perception styles can motive elevated anxiety and despair, that might in addition exacerbate physical symptoms of strain. Additionally, people who enjoy continual strain can also engage in risky behaviors, along facet overeating or substance abuse, which could further exacerbate bodily symptoms and signs and symptoms of pressure.

On the opportunity hand, individuals who have strong Psychological Immunity can be better capable of deal with stress and adversity, major to superior bodily and highbrow fitness outcomes. The thoughts-frame connection plays a critical function in this technique, as our thoughts, feelings, and behaviors can help us deal with stress and adversity.

For instance, human beings who've strong Psychological Immunity may additionally additionally engage in wholesome coping strategies, along with exercise, meditation, or social useful resource. These healthy coping strategies can help alleviate bodily signs and symptoms of strain and beautify intellectual fitness results. Additionally, humans who've sturdy Psychological Immunity also can moreover have top notch concept patterns, which encompass optimism or resilience, which could assist them deal with stress and adversity.

The mind-frame connection moreover plays a vital role within the improvement and manage of intellectual health troubles. Mental fitness issues, which consist of tension and despair, could have a high-quality impact on our physical fitness. For example, folks who experience anxiety may additionally have extended coronary coronary coronary heart charge, muscle anxiety, and adjustments in breathing. These bodily signs and symptoms and signs can exacerbate mental health symptoms, primary to a cycle of terrible bodily and intellectual fitness results.

The thoughts-body connection can also play a position inside the development of intellectual health troubles. For instance, those who enjoy chronic pressure may be at improved threat of developing tension or melancholy. Additionally, people who have experienced trauma can be at advanced chance of growing placed up-stressful pressure sickness (PTSD).

However, the thoughts-frame connection moreover may be used to control and deal with intellectual health troubles. For instance, folks who enjoy tension may additionally additionally gain from cognitive-behavioral therapy (CBT), which makes a speciality of converting horrible thought patterns and behaviors. Additionally, people who revel in depression might also moreover benefit from medication, that could assist alleviate physical signs and symptoms of despair.

In give up, the thoughts-frame connection plays a essential characteristic in Psychological Immunity and intellectual fitness outcomes. Our mind, feelings, and behaviors can have an effect on our bodily fitness, and vice versa. Chronic strain and adversity can motive numerous bodily and highbrow health issues, while healthy coping techniques and tremendous perception styles can improve intellectual and physical health results. The mind-body connection moreover performs a crucial feature inside the development and manipulate of highbrow health problems, highlighting the significance of early intervention and remedy. By understanding the mind-body connection, individuals can increase strong Psychological Immunity and enhance their normal health and well-being.

The Role of Exercise in Mental Health

The benefits of exercising on physical fitness are widely recognized, but the function of workout in highbrow health is regularly not noted. Exercise has been shown to have a exceptional effect on intellectual health, which consist of lowering signs and signs and symptoms and signs of melancholy and anxiety, enhancing mood, and improving cognitive feature. In this newsletter, we can discover the feature of workout in mental health and the mechanisms in the returned of its blessings.

Depression and Anxiety

Depression and tension are of the most commonplace intellectual health troubles, affecting tens of hundreds of thousands of humans international. Exercise has been tested to be an powerful remedy for each despair and tension. Studies have determined that workout can reduce signs of melancholy and tension, decorate temper, and boom feelings of well-being.

The mechanisms at the back of the blessings of exercise on melancholy and anxiety aren't absolutely understood, but there are numerous theories. One concept is that exercising will boom the producing of endorphins, that are herbal temper-boosting chemical materials inside the mind. Another principle is that exercising reduces infection within the frame, which has been linked to melancholy and anxiety.

In addition to those theories, exercising has additionally been proven to decorate self-esteem and social assist, which could have a first rate impact on mental fitness. Exercise can offer a experience of accomplishment and mastery, that might growth conceitedness. Exercise can also provide opportunities for social interplay, that may beautify social guide and reduce feelings of isolation.

Mood

Exercise has been validated to enhance mood, even in folks that do not have a recognized highbrow health ailment. Studies have located that exercising can beautify emotions of happiness, reduce feelings of pressure, and improve commonplace temper.

The mechanisms behind the advantages of exercising on temper are not in fact understood, but there are several theories.

One idea is that exercise increases the producing of endorphins, which might be natural temper-boosting chemical substances inside the mind. Another principle is that exercise reduces cortisol, that is a strain hormone which could have a terrible effect on mood.

In addition to the ones theories, exercise has moreover been validated to enhance sleep, that can have a great effect on mood. Exercise can help alter the sleep-wake cycle, principal to higher splendid sleep and advanced temper.

Cognitive Function

Exercise has been validated to beautify cognitive feature, which include memory, hobby, and executive characteristic. Studies have located that workout can decorate cognitive characteristic in each wholesome human beings and people with cognitive impairments.

The mechanisms inside the again of the blessings of workout on cognitive function aren't really understood, but there are numerous theories. One idea is that workout will growth blood waft to the mind, that could improve cognitive feature. Another idea is that exercising will growth the manufacturing of thoughts-derived neurotrophic factor (BDNF), that may be a protein that promotes the increase and survival of neurons inside the mind.

In addition to those theories, exercising has additionally been confirmed to reduce the risk of cognitive decline and dementia in older adults. Exercise can assist keep mind health and reduce the danger of cognitive impairments related to growing antique.

Conclusion: exercising has a powerful effect on intellectual health, which include lowering symptoms and signs and symptoms of depression and tension, enhancing mood, and enhancing cognitive characteristic. The mechanisms behind the blessings of exercise on intellectual fitness are not completely understood, however there are several theories. Exercise can increase the manufacturing of endorphins, lessen contamination, decorate vanity and social assist, alter the sleep-wake cycle, increase blood go together with the go with the flow to the mind, and growth the manufacturing of BDNF.

Despite the benefits of exercising on intellectual health, many humans with highbrow fitness issues do no longer engage in ordinary exercising. Barriers to exercise can consist of loss of motivation, loss of power, and absence of access to stable and less costly exercising facilities. Healthcare corporations can play a characteristic in promoting exercising as a remedy for highbrow health troubles and addressing boundaries to exercise.

In quit, workout is an powerful treatment for mental fitness issues and can have a awesome impact on temper, cognitive characteristic, and ordinary properly-being. By statistics the position of exercise in highbrow fitness, humans can contain workout into their treatment plan and decorate their intellectual health effects.

The Importance Of Sleep

Sleep is an important a part of our every day habitual, and it plays a critical role in retaining our bodily and highbrow fitness. While we sleep, our frame and mind go through a series of restorative techniques that assist us get over the stresses of the day and put together us for the annoying situations of tomorrow. In precise, sleep is essential for our Psychological Immunity , because it allows us adjust our feelings, consolidate our recollections, and improve our cognitive abilities.

One of the primary tactics that sleep permits our Psychological Immunity is thru regulating our emotions. When we're sleep-disadvantaged, we're much more likely to revel in poor emotions, inclusive of hysteria, irritability, and melancholy. This is because sleep deprivation disrupts the stability of neurotransmitters in our thoughts, which can be answerable for regulating our mood. In evaluation, at the same time as we get enough sleep, our mind is higher capable of adjust our emotions, allowing us to feel extra high quality and resilient in the face of pressure.

Another manner that sleep helps our Psychological Immunity is with the beneficial aid of consolidating our memories. During sleep, our mind techniques and stores the data that we've were given located out at some degree within the day, supporting us to keep critical information and overlook inappropriate facts. This method of memory consolidation is crucial for our cognitive functioning, because it allows us to research new talents, clear up issues, and make selections more effectively.

Finally, sleep is important for strengthening our cognitive skills, which includes hobby, popularity, and creativity. When we're sleep-disadvantaged, our cognitive normal overall performance suffers, as we have trouble focusing, making picks, and solving problems. In comparison, whilst we get enough sleep, our cognitive talents are greater appropriate, permitting us to anticipate greater surely, make higher options, and be greater cutting-edge in our questioning.

In end, sleep is a crucial element of our Psychological Immunity , because it lets in us regulate our feelings, consolidate our memories, and make stronger our cognitive talents. By prioritizing sleep in our every day routine, we are able to enhance our highbrow health and well-being, and be higher equipped to address the traumatic conditions of each day lifestyles.

## Chapter 2: Managing Stress And Anxiety

Understanding Stress and Anxiety

Stress and tension are  of the most common intellectual fitness troubles that humans face in recent times. They can be because of a choice of factors, which includes artwork-related pressure, financial concerns, courting issues, and fitness concerns. While stress and anxiety are normal responses to tough situations, they can end up complicated after they start to intrude with every day existence. In this text, we are able to find out the idea of know-how stress and tension in Psychological Immunity , and the way it is able to help human beings address those problems.

Stress and anxiety are often used interchangeably, however they're without a doubt  different things. Stress is a reaction to a hard situation, on the same time as tension is a enjoy of fear or unease about a few aspect that has now not but occurred. While pressure may be a superb force that motivates us to do so, anxiety can be a terrible stress that holds us again and prevents us from achieving our desires.

One of the critical issue additives of information stress and tension in Psychological Immunity is spotting the signs and signs and symptoms and signs of these situations. Stress can seem in loads of methods, collectively with bodily signs and symptoms together with headaches, muscle tension, and fatigue, in addition to emotional signs and symptoms which include irritability, mood swings, and problem concentrating. Anxiety, however, can motive bodily signs which consist of a racing heart, sweating, and trembling, further to emotional signs and signs and symptoms inclusive of fear, worry, and panic.

Another essential issue of know-how pressure and tension in Psychological Immunity is identifying the triggers that could cause those conditions to flare up. For a few human beings, pressure and anxiety may be brought about by using unique conditions, which incorporates public speakme or flying on an plane. For others, strain and anxiety can be extra generalized, and may be added about thru a selection of things, which consist of artwork-related pressure or monetary issues.

Once the symptoms and signs and symptoms of stress and tension had been identified, it is vital to broaden coping strategies to manipulate those situations. There are many precise strategies that can be used to manipulate pressure and tension, collectively with rest techniques which includes deep respiratory and meditation, exercise, and cognitive-behavioral remedy (CBT).

Relaxation strategies which encompass deep respiration and meditation can be effective in decreasing stress and tension with the aid of calming the mind and body. These strategies may be practiced at domestic or in a quiet area, and can be used each time strain or anxiety starts offevolved offevolved offevolved to feel overwhelming.

Exercise is some other effective way to control strain and anxiety. Exercise releases endorphins, which is probably herbal chemical compounds that assist to reduce stress and enhance temper. Exercise also can assist to beautify sleep, this is crucial for regular mental fitness and properly-being.

Cognitive-behavioral remedy (CBT) is a shape of speak remedy that can be used to assist people manipulate stress and tension. CBT makes a speciality of changing horrific concept styles and behaviors that could contribute to stress and anxiety. By figuring out and difficult awful thoughts, people can learn how to control their strain and tension in a more excessive great way.

In addition to those techniques, there also are lifestyle adjustments that may be made to assist manipulate strain and tension. These encompass getting enough sleep, ingesting a wholesome food regimen, and fending off alcohol and drugs. It is also important to workout accurate self-care, together with taking time for oneself and appealing in sports that convey pride and rest.

In stop, understanding strain and anxiety in Psychological Immunity is an essential element of preserving suitable intellectual fitness and properly-being. By recognizing the symptoms and signs and symptoms of those situations, identifying triggers, and growing coping techniques, humans can discover ways to control their stress and anxiety in a greater excellent way. Whether via relaxation techniques, workout, or cognitive-behavioral treatment, there are various splendid techniques that can be used to manipulate stress and anxiety and enhance fashionable mental fitness.

The Impact of Chronic Stress

Chronic pressure is a shape of strain that takes region over a prolonged time body. It can be because of a selection of factors, collectively with artwork-related strain, financial troubles, relationship problems, and fitness problems. While pressure is a regular a part of existence, chronic pressure may want to have a giant impact on highbrow health. In this article, we will discover the impact of persistent pressure on intellectual fitness, and the manner it could have an effect on people over time.

One of the critical issue components of knowledge the impact of chronic pressure on intellectual fitness is recognizing the signs and signs and symptoms and symptoms of persistent pressure. Chronic strain can take place in a number of strategies, together with physical symptoms and signs and signs and symptoms along side headaches, muscle tension, and fatigue, further to emotional signs and signs and symptoms together with irritability, mood swings, and problem concentrating. Chronic stress can also bring about behavioral changes, along with elevated alcohol or drug use, social withdrawal, and modifications in eating behavior.

Chronic strain should have a giant impact on intellectual fitness over the years. One of the maximum commonplace intellectual fitness problems related to chronic pressure is tension. Anxiety is a feeling of worry or unease approximately some thing that has not but came about, and it is able to be because of a variety of things, collectively with persistent stress. Chronic stress can also motive depression, that is a mood disease characterised thru the use of persistent emotions of unhappiness, hopelessness, and loss of hobby in sports activities that have been as quickly as a laugh.

In addition to anxiety and depression, chronic stress also can motive other intellectual health troubles, at the side of positioned up-disturbing pressure contamination (PTSD) and obsessive-compulsive ailment (OCD). PTSD is a intellectual fitness scenario that can upward push up after experiencing or witnessing a stressful occasion, and persistent pressure can boom the danger of growing PTSD. OCD is a intellectual health scenario characterised thru obsessive mind and compulsive behaviors, and continual stress can exacerbate symptoms and signs of OCD.

Chronic pressure also can have a huge effect on physical fitness. Chronic pressure can bring about some of physical health troubles, along with high blood strain, coronary heart illness, and weight issues. Chronic strain can also weaken the immune device, making human beings greater liable to illnesses and infections.

One of the reasons that chronic pressure may additionally need to have this sort of top notch impact on mental and physical fitness is that it can cause a country of continual infection. Chronic infection is a kind of infection that takes region over a extended time body, and it can purpose plenty of health issues, which incorporates highbrow health troubles which incorporates depression and anxiety. Chronic irritation also can purpose bodily health troubles together with coronary coronary heart disease and diabetes.

Another reason that continual strain can have the form of giant impact on highbrow fitness is that it can cause changes in mind shape and feature. Chronic strain can motive adjustments inside the mind's shape and feature, at the side of changes inside the duration and interest of the amygdala, that is the a part of the brain that is liable for processing feelings. Chronic stress can also cause modifications inside the hippocampus, it really is the a part of the mind that is liable for memory and gaining knowledge of.

In addition to the ones changes in mind shape and function, chronic pressure can also result in adjustments within the ranges of neurotransmitters in the mind. Neurotransmitters are chemicals that transmit alerts among neurons within the brain, and chronic stress can result in adjustments within the ranges of neurotransmitters together with serotonin and dopamine. These changes in neurotransmitter stages can motive highbrow fitness issues along with depression and anxiety.

In end, chronic stress ought to have a large effect on intellectual fitness through the years. Chronic strain can result in intellectual fitness problems consisting of hysteria, depression, PTSD, and OCD, in addition to physical fitness problems which includes excessive blood stress, coronary coronary coronary heart illness, and weight problems. Chronic stress can also result in adjustments in brain shape and feature, in addition to modifications in neurotransmitter tiers inside the mind. It is critical to recognize the signs and symptoms and signs and symptoms and symptoms and signs and signs and symptoms of persistent pressure, and to take steps to govern stress in a wholesome way that allows you to maintain pinnacle highbrow and physical fitness.

Cognitive-Behavioral Therapy Techniques

Cognitive-behavioral treatment (CBT) is a form of psychotherapy this is based on the idea that our thoughts, feelings, and behaviors are all interconnected. CBT strategies are designed to help humans grow to be aware of and task bad concept styles and behaviors which is probably contributing to their highbrow health issues. The aim of CBT is to help people growth greater best and adaptive processes of questioning and behaving, which can reason advanced mental health results.

CBT has been showed to be an effective remedy for a considerable form of highbrow health conditions, which encompass anxiety issues, depression, positioned up-stressful pressure infection (PTSD), obsessive-compulsive disease (OCD), and ingesting problems. CBT is frequently carried out in mixture with medication, in particular for human beings with more immoderate highbrow fitness issues. However, CBT also can be used as a standalone treatment for plenty intellectual fitness conditions, especially for people with slight to mild signs and symptoms and signs.

One of the vital element techniques applied in CBT is cognitive restructuring. This technique includes identifying and difficult negative idea patterns that contribute to intellectual fitness problems. For example, people with tension troubles can also will be inclined to catastrophize, or recollect the worst-case scenario in any given state of affairs. Cognitive restructuring consists of supporting human beings to find out the ones horrific concept patterns and replace them with more fantastic and practical mind.

Another crucial method utilized in CBT is exposure treatment. This method is often used to treat tension troubles and consists of little by little exposing people to the conditions or devices that cause their tension. The cause of publicity remedy is to assist human beings take a look at that the ones conditions or items are not simply dangerous, and to reduce their anxiety reaction over the years.

Behavioral activation is each different technique utilized in CBT. This approach entails assisting humans to pick out and interact in sports activities which is probably captivating and worthwhile, no matter the reality that they do no longer experience like doing them. This can be specially beneficial for humans with melancholy, who may additionally moreover have lost hobby in sports activities they as soon as loved.

Other CBT strategies encompass rest education, problem-solving skills schooling, and social abilities education. Relaxation schooling includes training individuals strategies which consist of deep respiration and present day muscle rest to help them manage their stress and anxiety. Problem-fixing skills schooling entails schooling individuals a way to find out and treatment issues of their lives in a extra effective manner. Social talents training consists of helping humans to beautify their conversation and interpersonal abilities, which can be specially beneficial for humans with social anxiety illness.

CBT is a pretty primarily based shape of psychotherapy, with a specific set of goals and techniques which may be used to assist humans manage their intellectual health signs and symptoms. CBT generally includes weekly or bi-weekly intervals with a professional therapist, and can final for severa months or longer, relying on the individual's goals.

## Chapter 3: Overcoming Depression

Defining Depression

Depression is a highbrow fitness illness that influences tens of millions of humans worldwide. It is characterized with the useful resource of the use of continual feelings of disappointment, hopelessness, and a loss of hobby in activities which have been once thrilling. Depression can be because of a selection of things, collectively with genetics, environmental factors, and life occasions.

Symptoms of melancholy can range from individual to character, however a few common signs embody a chronic low temper, emotions of worthlessness or guilt, hassle snoozing or oversleeping, changes in urge for food or weight, and a loss of electricity or motivation. In immoderate instances, melancholy can result in suicidal thoughts or behaviors.

Depression is a complicated situation that can be hard to apprehend and deal with. However, research has mounted that a aggregate of drugs, remedy, and way of lifestyles adjustments may be effective in managing signs and enhancing everyday satisfactory of lifestyles.

One of the maximum common styles of despair is crucial depressive illness (MDD), it is characterized with the resource of the use of continual feelings of unhappiness or a lack of interest in lifestyles. MDD may be because of a selection of things, which incorporates genetics, mind chemistry, and life events collectively with trauma or stress.

Another sort of despair is seasonal affective sickness (SAD), that could be a form of depression that occurs at some stage in the wintry weather months when there may be tons less daylight. SAD is idea to be due to a lack of sunlight, that could disrupt the body's inner clock and bring about modifications in temper and electricity levels.

Depression can also be because of unique clinical situations, which include thyroid problems or persistent pain. In the ones instances, treating the underlying clinical circumstance can assist beautify signs and symptoms and symptoms of melancholy.

While melancholy may be a tough circumstance to stay with, there are various sources available to help individuals manipulate their signs and symptoms and decorate their common first-class of life. Seeking professional assist from a intellectual health provider may be an crucial step in getting the guide and remedy had to manipulate depression. Additionally, making lifestyle adjustments consisting of getting regular workout, consuming a wholesome weight loss program, and training strain control techniques additionally can be useful in dealing with signs and signs of despair.

The Causes and Symptoms of Depression

Depression is a intellectual fitness ailment that affects thousands and thousands of people global. It is characterized through chronic feelings of unhappiness, hopelessness, and a lack of hobby in activities which have been as quickly as a laugh. Depression can be due to a desire of things, inclusive of genetics, environmental factors, and lifestyles activities.

Symptoms of melancholy can variety from character to character, but a few commonplace symptoms and signs and symptoms encompass a continual low mood, feelings of worthlessness or guilt, trouble sound asleep or oversleeping, adjustments in urge for meals or weight, and a loss of energy or motivation. In excessive instances, melancholy can result in suicidal thoughts or behaviors.

Depression is a complex situation that can be hard to apprehend and deal with. However, studies has verified that a mixture of drugs, remedy, and way of existence modifications can be powerful in handling signs and signs and symptoms and signs and symptoms and symptoms and improving common first-rate of life.

One of the maximum not unusual forms of despair is foremost depressive sickness (MDD), which is characterised through persistent emotions of sadness or a loss of hobby in existence. MDD may be because of a range of factors, together with genetics, mind chemistry, and life sports which encompass trauma or stress.

Another form of depression is seasonal affective ailment (SAD), it actually is a form of melancholy that happens in the direction of the iciness months while there can be a whole lot much less daytime. SAD is idea to be due to a lack of daylight hours, that may disrupt the frame's inner clock and cause changes in mood and energy tiers.

Depression moreover can be due to special clinical conditions, together with thyroid troubles or continual ache. In those instances, treating the underlying clinical situation can help enhance symptoms of despair.

While depression can be a difficult state of affairs to stay with, there are numerous sources to be had to help people manipulate their symptoms and signs and enhance their average top notch of life. Seeking professional help from a intellectual fitness company may be an important step in getting the guide and treatment needed to manipulate despair. Additionally, making manner of existence adjustments which encompass getting normal exercising, consuming a healthy eating regimen, and working closer to stress management strategies moreover may be useful in coping with symptoms of melancholy.

There are many capacity motives of melancholy, which incorporates genetic, environmental, and intellectual factors. Some of the most common causes of despair encompass:

1. Genetics: Research has proven that depression can run in households, suggesting that there may be a genetic detail to the sickness. Studies have recognized specific

genes that can be associated with an accelerated hazard of melancholy.

2. Brain chemistry: Depression is idea to be because of an imbalance of chemical compounds within the thoughts, which encompass serotonin and dopamine. These chemical materials are responsible for regulating temper, and even as they'll be out of stability, it may bring about symptoms and symptoms of despair.

three. Environmental elements: Life occasions together with trauma, strain, or loss can cause despair in some people. Additionally, living in a disturbing or chaotic surroundings can growth the chance of developing depression.

four. Medical conditions: Certain scientific situations, collectively with thyroid problems or continual pain, can growth the chance of growing melancholy. Additionally, medicinal drugs used to address the ones conditions can every now and then motive despair as a aspect effect.

five. Substance abuse: Substance abuse can increase the chance of growing melancholy, as drugs and alcohol can disrupt thoughts chemistry and bring about changes in mood and behavior.

The symptoms of depression can range from man or woman to individual, but some commonplace signs and symptoms include:

1. Persistent low temper: Individuals with melancholy may also moreover experience sad, hopeless, or empty for extended periods of time.

2. Loss of hobby: Individuals with depression may also get bored in sports they as soon as cherished, which includes interests or socializing.

3. Changes in urge for meals or weight: Depression can reason modifications in urge for food, most important to weight advantage or weight loss.

4. Sleep disturbances: Depression can cause trouble drowsing or oversleeping.

5. Fatigue: Individuals with despair may also revel in tired or lack power, even as soon as you've got enough sleep.

6. Feelings of worthlessness or guilt: Depression can reason human beings to revel in nugatory or accountable, even when there can be no logical motive for those feelings.

7. Difficulty concentrating: Depression must make it hard to pay attention or make selections.

eight. Suicidal thoughts or behaviors: In excessive instances, depression can cause suicidal thoughts or behaviors.

Overall, melancholy is a complicated state of affairs that may be due to a selection of things. Seeking expert assist from a intellectual health company can be an important step in getting the guide and remedy needed to manipulate despair. Additionally, making way of existence adjustments which includes getting regular exercising, ingesting a healthful food regimen, and schooling stress manipulate strategies additionally may be beneficial in managing symptoms and symptoms of melancholy.

Evidence-Based Treatments for Depression

Depression is a not unusual highbrow health disease that impacts hundreds of thousands of human beings worldwide. It is characterized with the useful useful resource of emotions of sadness, hopelessness, and a lack of interest in sports activities that have been as soon as exciting. Depression can be because of a selection of things, including genetics, environmental elements, and existence occasions. It is a complex sickness that calls for an entire method to remedy. Evidence-based treatments for despair are those that have been scientifically tested and examined to be effective in treating depression. In this newsletter, we're able to discover the severa evidence-based totally completely remedies for depression.

Cognitive Behavioral Therapy (CBT)

Cognitive Behavioral Therapy (CBT) is a form of communicate treatment that specializes in converting horrible idea styles and behaviors that contribute to depression. CBT is primarily based completely on the concept that our thoughts, feelings, and behaviors are interconnected. By converting our mind and behaviors, we're able to alternate how we enjoy. CBT is a quick-term therapy that commonly lasts among 12 and 20 classes. During CBT, the therapist works with the affected character to find out lousy perception patterns and behaviors and extend strategies to change them. CBT has been set up to be powerful in treating depression, with studies displaying that it's miles as powerful as medicine in treating mild to mild melancholy.

Interpersonal Therapy (IPT)

Interpersonal Therapy (IPT) is a shape of speak treatment that makes a speciality of improving interpersonal relationships and communique talents. IPT is primarily based on the concept that melancholy is frequently as a result of interpersonal issues, along with conflicts with own family contributors or pals. During IPT, the therapist works with the patient to select out out and cope with those interpersonal problems. IPT is a short-term remedy that generally lasts among 12 and sixteen intervals. Studies have demonstrated that IPT is powerful in treating depression, particularlyDepression is a common highbrow fitness ailment that impacts hundreds of thousands of humans worldwide. It is characterised with the useful resource of continual feelings of sadness, hopelessness, and a lack of interest in sports which have been as soon as amusing. Depression can be on account of a range of factors, at the side of genetics, environmental factors, and lifestyles sports activities. It can be a debilitating situation that affects a person's capability to characteristic of their every day existence. Fortunately, there are evidence-primarily based totally treatments available which could assist people manipulate their symptoms and symptoms and beautify their first rate of life.

The first-line treatment for melancholy is psychotherapy, moreover called communicate remedy. Psychotherapy includes meeting with a intellectual health expert to talk approximately your mind, feelings, and behaviors. There are numerous kinds of psychotherapy which have been examined to be effective in treating depression, which include cognitive-behavioral remedy (CBT), interpersonal remedy (IPT), and psychodynamic remedy.

Cognitive-behavioral remedy (CBT) is a shape of psychotherapy that makes a speciality of converting terrible perception patterns and behaviors that contribute to depression. CBT is primarily based on the idea that our mind, emotions, and behaviors are interconnected, and that converting you will result in adjustments within the others. In CBT, human beings paintings with a therapist to end up aware of awful idea styles and learn

41

techniques to update them with greater fantastic and practical mind. CBT has been established to be effective in treating melancholy, with studies displaying that it can be as effective as remedy for moderate to mild despair.

Interpersonal treatment (IPT) is a form of psychotherapy that focuses on enhancing interpersonal relationships and communique talents. IPT is primarily based definitely at the idea that melancholy can be because of issues in relationships with others, and that improving these relationships can bring about upgrades in temper. In IPT, individuals art work with a therapist to come to be privy to and address interpersonal troubles, collectively with conflicts with own family humans or buddies. IPT has been proven to be effective in treating melancholy, particularly in people with interpersonal troubles.

Psychodynamic therapy is a type of psychotherapy that specializes in exploring unconscious thoughts and emotions that may be contributing to depression. Psychodynamic remedy is primarily based completely mostly on the concept that our early studies and relationships can shape our current mind, feelings, and behaviors. In psychodynamic remedy, humans paintings with a therapist to find out their past studies and the way they'll be impacting their modern mood. Psychodynamic treatment has been demonstrated to be powerful in treating despair, mainly in humans with a statistics of trauma or young people stressors.

In addition to psychotherapy, treatment is frequently used to deal with depression. Antidepressant drug treatments artwork with the resource of way of changing the levels of tremendous chemical compounds within the thoughts, on the side of serotonin and norepinephrine. There are severa types of antidepressant medicinal tablets to be had, which includes selective serotonin reuptake inhibitors (SSRIs), serotonin-norepinephrine reuptake inhibitors (SNRIs), and tricyclic antidepressants (TCAs). Antidepressant drug treatments can be powerful in treating depression, particularly in people with mild to severe despair.

Another proof-based remedy for despair is electroconvulsive treatment (ECT). ECT entails passing an electrical present day-day through the mind to bring about a seizure. ECT is usually utilized in people with excessive despair who have no longer spoke back to other treatments. ECT has been tested to be powerful in treating despair, with research displaying that it is able to be as effective as medication for excessive melancholy.

Finally, there are numerous possibility treatments for depression which have tested promise in studies studies. These consist of exercise, mindfulness-based totally definitely absolutely treatment alternatives, and slight remedy. Exercise has been showed to be effective in decreasing signs and symptoms of melancholy, with research showing that it can be as powerful as treatment for mild to mild despair. Mindfulness-primarily based treatments, which includes mindfulness-based completely cognitive remedy (MBCT), have moreover been hooked up to be powerful in treating despair, specifically in individuals with a information of recurrent despair. Light treatment includes exposure to bright mild, typically in the morning, and has been proven to be effective in treating seasonal affective sickness (SAD), a shape of depression that happens at some point of the winter months.

## Chapter 4: Coping With Trauma And Ptsd

Understanding Trauma and PTSD

Trauma is a great sized event or series of events that could have a protracted-lasting effect on an man or woman's highbrow and emotional properly-being. Trauma can be due to a whole lot of reviews, which includes bodily or sexual abuse, natural screw ups, accidents, violence, or army combat. Trauma can purpose severa intellectual fitness problems, which include put up-annoying pressure sickness (PTSD). In this newsletter, we are able to discover the character of trauma, the signs and symptoms and symptoms and signs and symptoms and symptoms of PTSD, and the treatment options available for the ones who've skilled trauma.

What is Trauma?

Trauma is a complex and subjective experience which could have a profound effect on an individual's lifestyles. Trauma may be due to a whole lot of research, together with:

Physical or sexual abuse

Natural disasters

Accidents

Violence

Military fight

Witnessing or experiencing a lifestyles-threatening event

Trauma could have a protracted-lasting impact on an man or woman's highbrow and emotional properly-being. Trauma can result in various highbrow fitness problems, together with anxiety, depression, and PTSD.

What is PTSD?

PTSD is a highbrow fitness illness that could extend after an character has professional or witnessed a demanding occasion. PTSD can increase after a unmarried traumatic occasion or after repeated publicity to trauma. PTSD may also have a terrific impact on an character's each day existence, making it hard to function commonly.

Symptoms of PTSD

The symptoms and symptoms of PTSD can range from person to character and might growth at any time after the worrying occasion. The signs and symptoms and symptoms of PTSD may be grouped into 4 classes:

1. Intrusive Thoughts and Memories

Intrusive mind and recollections are one of the hallmark signs of PTSD. Individuals with PTSD may additionally furthermore revel in vivid and distressing memories of the annoying event. These recollections may be added approximately through way of an entire lot of stimuli, together with elements of hobby, sounds, and smells. Individuals with PTSD can also revel in nightmares or flashbacks of the demanding occasion.

2. Avoidance

Individuals with PTSD also can keep away from people, places, or subjects that remind them of the worrying occasion. This avoidance can make it hard to interact in ordinary every day activities, which includes going to artwork or faculty.

three. Negative Changes in Mood and Cognition

PTSD can reason horrific changes in temper and cognition. Individuals with PTSD might also additionally revel in emotions of guilt, disgrace, or hopelessness. They might also furthermore have trouble remembering important statistics about the traumatic event or have a negative outlook at the destiny.

four. Hyperarousal

Hyperarousal is a state of heightened alertness which can make it hard to lighten up or sleep. Individuals with PTSD may be effortlessly startled or enjoy on side. They can also have problem concentrating or experience irritability or anger.

Treatment for PTSD

PTSD is a treatable state of affairs, and there are several remedy options available for humans who've expert trauma. The best remedy for PTSD is psychotherapy, that might assist people method the annoying occasion and growth coping strategies to control symptoms and symptoms and symptoms.

1. Cognitive Behavioral Therapy (CBT)

CBT is a kind of psychotherapy that specializes in converting horrific idea styles and behaviors. CBT can help humans with PTSD pick out and project horrible thoughts related to the disturbing occasion. CBT can also help people boom coping techniques to manipulate symptoms of PTSD.

2. Eye Movement Desensitization and Reprocessing (EMDR)

EMDR is a shape of psychotherapy that consists of guided eye movements on the identical time because the man or woman recollects the traumatic occasion. EMDR can assist individuals machine the stressful event and reduce the intensity of intrusive mind and reminiscences.

three. Medication

Medication can be used to control signs of PTSD, which encompass tension, melancholy, and insomnia. Antidepressants and anti-anxiety medicines are generally used to address PTSD.

four. Group Therapy

Group remedy can be an effective treatment opportunity for humans with PTSD. Group remedy can provide a supportive environment for human beings to percentage their reviews and growth coping strategies.

five. Self-Care

Self-care is an critical part of dealing with signs and symptoms of PTSD. Engaging in activities that sell rest and properly-being, which includes exercise, meditation, or spending time in nature, can help lessen signs and signs and symptoms and symptoms and signs and symptoms of PTSD.

In end, trauma is a big event or series of sports that could have an enduring effect on an man or woman's intellectual and emotional properly-being. PTSD is a intellectual fitness disease that can extend after an individual has skilled or witnessed a annoying event. The signs and symptoms and signs of PTSD may be grouped into 4 education: intrusive mind and memories, avoidance, horrible modifications in temper and cognition, and hyperarousal. PTSD is a treatable scenario, and there are various remedy alternatives to be had, which incorporates psychotherapy, medicine, institution remedy, and self-care. If you or someone is experiencing signs of PTSD, it's far essential to are seeking out help from a highbrow health professional.

The Impact of Trauma on Mental Health

Trauma may moreover have a massive effect on an man or woman's intellectual health.

The impact of trauma on intellectual health can range from man or woman to individual and can rely on a choice of things, inclusive of the kind of trauma, the severity of the trauma, and the character's coping mechanisms.

## 1. Depression

Depression is a not unusual highbrow health problem that can boom after trauma. Individuals who have professional trauma may also additionally experience sad, hopeless, and feature a lack of hobby in sports activities activities they as soon as cherished. Depression could make it hard to characteristic typically and can have a great effect on an character's every day life.

## 2. Anxiety

Anxiety is a few special common highbrow fitness problem that would amplify after trauma. Individuals who've professional trauma can also enjoy worrying, worried, or on element. Anxiety ought to make it tough to loosen up or sleep and may interfere with each day sports sports.

three. Post-Traumatic Stress Disorder (PTSD)

PTSD is a intellectual fitness illness which could develop after an man or woman has experienced or witnessed a traumatic event. PTSD may have a large impact on an person's each day life, making it difficult to feature normally. The symptoms of PTSD may be grouped into 4 instructions: intrusive thoughts and recollections, avoidance, bad changes in temper and cognition, and hyperarousal.

4. Substance Abuse

Substance abuse is a common coping mechanism for human beings who've expert trauma. Substance abuse can provide temporary remedy from the symptoms of trauma, but can result in addiction and other terrible results.

5. Other Psychological Disorders

Trauma can also purpose awesome intellectual troubles, along side borderline man or woman disorder, dissociative issues, and consuming troubles. These issues may have a full-size effect on an man or woman's each day lifestyles and may require specialized treatment.

Treatment for Trauma

Trauma is a treatable circumstance, and there are numerous remedy alternatives to be had for human beings who have skilled trauma. The best treatment for trauma is psychotherapy, that could help human beings manner the disturbing occasion and increase coping strategies to control symptoms.

1. Cognitive Behavioral Therapy (CBT)

CBT is a shape of psychotherapy that specializes in changing terrible concept patterns and behaviors. CBT can help people with trauma pick out out and task terrible thoughts related to the disturbing occasion.

CBT can also help humans boom coping techniques to control signs of trauma.

2. Eye Movement Desensitization and Reprocessing (EMDR)

EMDR is a shape of psychotherapy that consists of guided eye movements even as the man or woman recalls the traumatic event. EMDR can help human beings technique the stressful occasion and decrease the depth of intrusive thoughts and memories.

three. Medication

Medication can be used to manipulate signs and symptoms of trauma, including despair, tension, and PTSD. Antidepressants and anti-tension medicines are normally used to deal with trauma.

four. Group Therapy

Group remedy can be an effective treatment choice for human beings with trauma. Group remedy can provide a supportive surroundings for humans to percent their reviews and extend coping techniques.

## 5. Self-Care

Self-care is an essential part of dealing with signs and signs and symptoms and symptoms and symptoms of trauma. Engaging in activities that sell rest and properly-being, which includes exercising, meditation, or spending time in nature, can assist lessen symptoms of trauma.

In cease, trauma is a massive occasion or collection of events that can have a long-lasting effect on an individual's intellectual and emotional well-being. Trauma can bring about pretty various intellectual health troubles, which embody melancholy, anxiety, PTSD, and special mental problems. The impact of trauma on highbrow health can variety from man or woman to man or woman and might rely on a choice of things. Trauma is a treatable situation, and there are numerous remedy options to be had, which encompass psychotherapy, medication, institution remedy, and self-care. If you or a person you understand is experiencing signs of trauma, it's far critical to are searching out help from a highbrow health professional.

Evidence-Based Treatments for PTSD

Post-traumatic pressure illness (PTSD) is a intellectual health state of affairs which could amplify after an person memories or witnesses a stressful occasion. PTSD can have a vast impact on an character's every day lifestyles, making it tough to function normally. Fortunately, there are several proof-based totally truely treatments to be had for PTSD that could help human beings control signs and symptoms and signs and symptoms and improve their first-rate of existence. In this text, we're able to discover the person of PTSD, the proof-primarily based without a doubt remedies to be had for PTSD, and the advantages and boundaries of these remedies.

What is PTSD?

PTSD is a highbrow fitness situation which can expand after an individual research or witnesses a worrying event. Traumatic activities can include physical or sexual assault, herbal disasters, injuries, violence, or navy combat. PTSD ought to have a big impact on an individual's every day lifestyles, making it difficult to function normally. The signs of PTSD may be grouped into four classes: intrusive mind and memories, avoidance, awful adjustments in mood and cognition, and hyperarousal.

## 1. Intrusive Thoughts and Memories

Individuals with PTSD can also moreover moreover enjoy intrusive mind and reminiscences associated with the traumatic event. These thoughts and reminiscences may be distressing and may intervene with every day sports activities.

## 2. Avoidance

Individuals with PTSD can also keep away from situations or activities that remind them of the worrying occasion. Avoidance must make it difficult to have interaction in regular each day sports and might result in social isolation.

3. Negative Changes in Mood and Cognition

Individuals with PTSD also can experience terrible changes in temper and cognition, together with emotions of guilt, disgrace, or hopelessness. They also can have trouble remembering or focusing on duties.

4. Hyperarousal

Individuals with PTSD may additionally revel in hyperarousal, that might embody being with out problems startled, feeling on element, or having hassle sleeping. Hyperarousal can make it tough to loosen up and can intrude with every day sports sports.

Evidence-Based Treatments for PTSD

There are numerous evidence-based totally completely remedies available for PTSD that have been set up to be effective in dealing with symptoms and signs and enhancing fine of life. The best remedies for PTSD are psychotherapies, that might assist individuals way the worrying event and develop coping strategies to control symptoms.

1. Cognitive Behavioral Therapy (CBT)

CBT is a shape of psychotherapy that makes a speciality of converting bad concept patterns and behaviors. CBT can help humans with PTSD find out and mission terrible thoughts related to the demanding event. CBT can also assist humans expand coping strategies to manipulate symptoms of PTSD.

2. Prolonged Exposure Therapy (PE)

PE is a type of psychotherapy that consists of step by step exposing people with PTSD to the recollections and situations that reason their signs and symptoms. PE can help individuals approach the annoying occasion and decrease the intensity of intrusive thoughts and reminiscences.

three. Eye Movement Desensitization and Reprocessing (EMDR)

EMDR is a form of psychotherapy that consists of guided eye movements on the identical time as the individual remembers the stressful occasion. EMDR can help people machine the annoying event and decrease the intensity of intrusive thoughts and reminiscences.

four. Cognitive Processing Therapy (CPT)

CPT is a shape of psychotherapy that specializes in supporting humans with PTSD assignment and trade horrible mind associated with the annoying event. CPT can assist individuals boom coping strategies to govern symptoms and symptoms and signs and symptoms of PTSD.

5. Medication

Medication may be used to govern signs and symptoms and signs of PTSD, which incorporates despair, anxiety, and hyperarousal. Antidepressants and anti-anxiety medicines are usually used to cope with PTSD.

Benefits and Limitations of Evidence-Based Treatments for PTSD

Evidence-primarily based treatments for PTSD may be powerful in handling signs and symptoms and enhancing exceptional of existence. However, those remedies have obstacles and might not paintings for anyone.

1. Effectiveness

Evidence-primarily based treatments for PTSD were proven to be effective in coping with symptoms and improving brilliant of existence. However, the effectiveness of these treatments can vary from individual to individual and may rely upon a desire of factors, together with the severity of the trauma, the man or woman's coping mechanisms, and the individual's willingness to have interaction in remedy.

2. Time Commitment

Evidence-based completely completely treatments for PTSD can be time-ingesting and require a widespread dedication from the person. Psychotherapies for PTSD can require severa months of weekly sessions, and medication may also moreover want to be taken for an prolonged time frame.

3. Side Effects

Medications used to address PTSD need to have aspect results, along side drowsiness, dizziness, and nausea. These difficulty results can intervene with every day sports activities and may require the person to regulate their remedy or dosage.

4. Stigma

There remains a stigma associated with looking for remedy for intellectual health conditions, which includes PTSD. This stigma can also want to make it hard for people to are searching for treatment and may purpose emotions of shame or embarrassment.

In quit, PTSD is a highbrow fitness situation that could increase after an character critiques or witnesses a annoying event. There are numerous evidence-based totally absolutely truely remedies to be had for PTSD that would help individuals manage symptoms and signs and symptoms and signs and symptoms and enhance their fantastic of life. The best remedies for PTSD are psychotherapies, collectively with CBT, PE, EMDR, and CPT. Medication also can be used to govern signs and symptoms and symptoms and signs and symptoms of PTSD. These treatments have benefits and limitations and may not paintings for truely everyone. If you or a person you recognize is experiencing signs of PTSD, it's far vital to are trying to find assist from a intellectual fitness expert.

The Role of Medication in Treating PTSD

Post-worrying stress sickness (PTSD) is a intellectual fitness scenario which could growth after an person reviews or witnesses a annoying event. PTSD may additionally have a big effect on an individual's each day existence, making it difficult to feature commonly. While psychotherapies are the extremely good remedies for PTSD, treatment also can play a function in coping with symptoms and symptoms. In this article, we're able to explore the location of drugs in treating PTSD, which encompass the types of treatment used, their effectiveness, and their capability facet consequences.

Types of Medication Used to Treat PTSD

There are numerous sorts of remedy that may be used to deal with PTSD, along side antidepressants, anti-anxiety medicinal tablets, and antipsychotics.

1. Antidepressants

Antidepressants are commonly used to address symptoms and signs and symptoms and signs and symptoms of PTSD, together with despair, anxiety, and insomnia. Selective serotonin reuptake inhibitors (SSRIs) are the most generally prescribed antidepressants for

PTSD. SSRIs artwork by growing the degrees of serotonin within the thoughts, which could enhance temper and decrease anxiety.

2. Anti-Anxiety Medications

Anti-anxiety medicinal capsules, additionally referred to as anxiolytics, are used to treat symptoms and signs of anxiety, which encompass panic assaults, agitation, and hyperarousal. Benzodiazepines are the most usually prescribed anti-anxiety medicinal pills for PTSD. Benzodiazepines paintings through enhancing the effects of a neurotransmitter referred to as gamma-aminobutyric acid (GABA), that would lessen tension and promote relaxation.

3. Antipsychotics

Antipsychotics are once in a while used to treat symptoms and symptoms and symptoms of PTSD, together with hallucinations, delusions, and paranoia. Atypical antipsychotics are the maximum normally prescribed antipsychotics for PTSD.

Atypical antipsychotics art work through blocking off dopamine receptors within the mind, that may reduce hallucinations and delusions.

Effectiveness of Medication in Treating PTSD

Medication may be powerful in dealing with signs and symptoms of PTSD, at the side of despair, anxiety, and hyperarousal. However, the effectiveness of medicine can range from character to man or woman and can depend upon a variety of factors, along with the severity of the trauma, the person's coping mechanisms, and the character's willingness to interact in treatment.

1. Antidepressants

Antidepressants have been proven to be powerful in dealing with signs of PTSD, which incorporates melancholy, tension, and insomnia. SSRIs are the maximum usually prescribed antidepressants for PTSD and have been validated to be effective in decreasing signs and symptoms of PTSD in numerous medical trials. However, the effectiveness of SSRIs can variety from individual to individual and might take numerous weeks to turn out to be fundamental.

2. Anti-Anxiety Medications

Anti-tension medicines may be powerful in coping with signs and symptoms of tension, which incorporates panic assaults, agitation, and hyperarousal. Benzodiazepines are the most normally prescribed anti-anxiety drug remedies for PTSD and were validated to be powerful in reducing signs and symptoms and signs and symptoms of PTSD in several medical trials. However, benzodiazepines may be addiction-forming and can reason drowsiness, dizziness, and confusion.

three. Antipsychotics

Antipsychotics can be effective in dealing with signs and symptoms and symptoms and signs and symptoms of PTSD, collectively with hallucinations, delusions, and paranoia. Atypical antipsychotics are the maximum typically prescribed antipsychotics for PTSD and had been established to be powerful in lowering signs and symptoms and signs and symptoms of PTSD in severa scientific trials. However, bizarre antipsychotics can motive component effects, which include weight advantage, diabetes, and movement issues.

Potential Side Effects of Medication for PTSD

Medication used to address PTSD can reason facet results, consisting of drowsiness, dizziness, nausea, and sexual sickness. The facet effects of medication can intervene with every day activities and might require the man or woman to alter their remedy or dosage.

1. Antidepressants

Antidepressants can purpose factor consequences, which includes drowsiness, dizziness, nausea, and sexual ailment. These factor effects can intrude with each day sports sports and can require the individual to modify their remedy or dosage. In uncommon instances, antidepressants can purpose suicidal mind or behavior, especially in youngsters and young adults.

2. Anti-Anxiety Medications

Anti-tension medicines can motive element consequences, which include drowsiness, dizziness, confusion, and reminiscence issues. These issue effects can intrude with every day sports sports and may require the man or woman to regulate their remedy or dosage. Benzodiazepines also can be dependancy-forming and can motive withdrawal signs if stopped .

three. Antipsychotics

Antipsychotics can cause factor results, which embody drowsiness, dizziness, weight advantage, diabetes, and movement issues. These side effects can intervene with every day sports activities and can require the person to adjust their remedy or dosage. Atypical antipsychotics also can growth the danger of stroke and lack of lifestyles in elderly people with dementia.

Limitations of Medication for PTSD

Medication can be powerful in managing signs of PTSD, but it isn't always a remedy for the situation. Medication also can have boundaries and might not artwork for absolutely everybody.

1. Effectiveness

The effectiveness of medicine for PTSD can variety from individual to individual and may rely on a selection of things, which incorporates the severity of the trauma, the individual's coping mechanisms, and the person's willingness to engage in treatment.

# Chapter 5: Navigating Relationships And Social Support

The Importance of Social Support

Building strong relationships is an vital detail of Psychological Immunity . Relationships are a crucial a part of human existence, and they may be able to have a large effect on our intellectual health and well-being. Strong relationships can offer us with emotional help, a enjoy of belonging, and a supply of motivation and concept. In this article, we are able to find out the importance of constructing sturdy relationships in Psychological Immunity and how it could assist human beings deal with emotional misery and intellectual damage.

Strong relationships can offer individuals with emotional useful resource, it really is critical in Psychological Immunity . Emotional help entails presenting consolation, empathy, and know-how to individuals who are going via hard instances. Strong relationships can offer people with a consistent and supportive surroundings wherein they could speak their intellectual health worries without worry of judgment or discrimination. This emotional help can assist humans deal with pressure, anxiety, and melancholy, and may provide them with the motivation and concept they need to overcome worrying situations.

Strong relationships can also provide humans with a sense of belonging, that is essential in Psychological Immunity . A experience of belonging includes feeling associated with others and feeling like you're a part of a community. This experience of belonging can help human beings revel in much less isolated and by myself, which can be a huge deliver of strain and tension. Strong relationships can offer humans with a feel of purpose and because of this, which can help them stay introduced on and targeted inside the course of difficult instances.

In addition to emotional resource and a enjoy of belonging, strong relationships can also provide human beings with a deliver of motivation and notion. Motivation and concept contain feeling energized and driven to advantage your dreams and pursue your passions. Strong relationships can offer individuals with the encouragement, motivation, and belongings they want to pursue their desires and desires. This can help people live targeted and inspired, although they will be going through demanding situations or setbacks.

Research has confirmed that sturdy relationships can have a substantial effect on intellectual fitness and nicely-being. Studies have located that human beings who have sturdy social resource networks are a whole lot much less likely to increase mental health problems, which consist of depression and tension. Strong relationships can also assist humans deal with strain and trauma. For example, people who have robust relationships after a annoying occasion, which includes a herbal disaster or a terrorist attack, generally generally generally tend to revel in a lot much less psychological distress and get better greater brief.

One of the key benefits of constructing strong relationships in Psychological Immunity is that it may help humans construct resilience. Resilience refers to the potential to get higher from difficult situations and overcome adversity. Individuals who have sturdy relationships have a tendency to be extra resilient and higher capable of deal with existence's disturbing conditions. Strong relationships can offer people with a experience of safety and balance, which could assist them stay grounded and focused within the course of tough times.

Building sturdy relationships also can help people develop healthy coping mechanisms. Coping mechanisms are the techniques that humans use to manipulate strain and emotional misery. Healthy coping mechanisms, which includes exercise, meditation, and remedy, can help people control pressure and decorate their intellectual health. Strong relationships can offer individuals with the encouragement, motivation, and assets they need to boom healthful coping mechanisms.

Another critical gain of constructing robust relationships in Psychological Immunity is that it can assist humans overcome stigma and discrimination. Stigma and discrimination can be big obstacles to looking for assist and assist for intellectual fitness problems. Strong relationships can offer human beings with a safe and supportive surroundings in which they are able to speak their intellectual health issues with out fear of judgment or discrimination. Strong relationships can also help humans challenge terrible stereotypes and attitudes approximately intellectual health.

Building sturdy relationships also can play a vital feature in stopping intellectual fitness problems. Studies have placed that people who have robust social assist networks are an entire lot a good deal much less probable to boom highbrow fitness troubles, which incorporates melancholy and tension. Strong relationships can provide people with the emotional and mental property they want to deal with pressure and different stressful situations before they become more critical highbrow health troubles.

Despite the various advantages of building strong relationships in Psychological Immunity , many people battle to assemble and maintain robust relationships. This may be due to a choice of factors, such as social isolation, stigma, and discrimination. It is critical for humans to take proactive steps to assemble and maintain strong relationships, together with turning into a member of golf equipment or businesses, volunteering, and conducting out to buddies and circle of relatives.

In stop, constructing robust relationships is a vital aspect of Psychological Immunity which could assist human beings deal with emotional misery and intellectual harm.

Strong relationships can provide human beings with emotional help, a enjoy of belonging, and a supply of motivation and concept. Building robust relationships also can help individuals construct resilience, increase healthful coping mechanisms, triumph over stigma and discrimination, and save you highbrow health troubles. It is crucial for people to take proactive steps to assemble and preserve robust relationships, as this may help them lead happier, extra healthful, and additional applicable lives

Building Strong Relationships

Social assist can play a crucial role in Psychological Immunity thru presenting human beings with the emotional and highbrow resources they need to deal with strain, trauma, and unique worrying conditions. Social aid can are available many forms, which incorporates emotional assist, informational resource, and tangible manual. Emotional manual includes supplying comfort, empathy, and statistics to folks that are going thru hard instances. Informational help entails supplying advice, guidance, and facts to individuals who need it. Tangible resource includes supplying sensible help, which includes financial help, transportation, or help with family chores.

Research has verified that social manual should have a extraordinary effect on intellectual fitness. Studies have located that people who have robust social guide networks are a amazing deal plenty less in all likelihood to increase intellectual health troubles, which includes despair and tension. Social manual can also help people address stress and trauma. For example, human beings who have social help after a disturbing event, which include a herbal disaster or a terrorist attack, commonly generally tend to enjoy tons less mental distress and get better more speedy.

One of the essential issue blessings of social help in Psychological Immunity is that it could help people construct resilience. Resilience refers to the capability to get higher from difficult situations and conquer adversity. Individuals who have sturdy social help networks will be predisposed to be more resilient and higher capable of deal with lifestyles's disturbing situations. Social useful resource can offer people with a experience of belonging, cause, and because of this, which could assist them stay stimulated and centered throughout difficult instances.

Social useful resource can also assist human beings boom healthy coping mechanisms. Coping mechanisms are the strategies that people use to govern strain and emotional misery. Healthy coping mechanisms, which includes workout, meditation, and remedy, can help people manage stress and decorate their highbrow health. Social assist can offer human beings with the encouragement, motivation, and assets they want to increase healthful coping mechanisms.

Another vital advantage of social manual in Psychological Immunity is that it can assist humans triumph over stigma and discrimination. Stigma and discrimination can be full-size barriers to looking for assist and guide for highbrow fitness troubles. Social help can offer people with a secure and supportive environment in which they are able to speak their intellectual health problems without worry of judgment or discrimination. Social manual can also help individuals mission awful stereotypes and attitudes approximately intellectual fitness.

Social assist also can play a critical feature in preventing highbrow fitness troubles. Studies have determined that human beings who've sturdy social help networks are much less likely to boom intellectual fitness problems, which includes melancholy and tension. Social assist can provide individuals with the emotional and psychological sources they need to deal with pressure and unique demanding conditions in advance than they emerge as more extreme highbrow health problems.

Despite the severa advantages of social resource in Psychological Immunity , many people battle to construct and preserve strong social help networks. This can be due to a selection of factors, which embody social isolation, stigma, and discrimination. It is vital for human beings to take proactive steps to construct and maintain social assist networks, inclusive of joining clubs or companies, volunteering, and engaging in out to pals and own family.

In give up, social resource is a vital element of Psychological Immunity that would help human beings deal with emotional distress and mental harm. Social aid can offer human beings with the emotional and intellectual assets they want to construct resilience, broaden healthy coping mechanisms, overcome stigma and discrimination, and save you highbrow health troubles. It is important for people to take proactive steps to construct and hold robust social assist networks, as this can assist them lead happier, healthier, and further pleasing lives.

The Impact of Toxic Relationships

Building robust relationships is an important factor of Psychological Immunity . Relationships are a vital a part of human life, and they may be capable of have a big impact on our highbrow health and nicely-being. Strong relationships can offer us with emotional resource, a sense of belonging, and a deliver of motivation and concept. In this newsletter, we're able to find out the significance of building robust relationships in Psychological Immunity and the way it could help humans cope with emotional misery and mental harm.

Strong relationships can offer human beings with emotional aid, it really is vital in Psychological Immunity . Emotional assist includes presenting comfort, empathy, and recognize-the way to folks that are going thru tough times. Strong relationships can offer human beings with a secure and supportive environment in which they are capable of talk their intellectual fitness problems without fear of judgment or discrimination. This emotional assist can help individuals deal with pressure, anxiety, and despair, and can provide them with the incentive and concept they need to triumph over disturbing conditions.

Strong relationships can also offer individuals with a feel of belonging, this is vital in Psychological Immunity . A experience of belonging includes feeling associated with others and feeling like you are a part of a community. This experience of belonging can help people feel less remoted and by myself, which may be a great supply of stress and tension. Strong relationships can provide people with a experience of motive and because of this, that might assist them live inspired and centered at some stage in difficult instances.

In addition to emotional assist and a revel in of belonging, strong relationships also can provide human beings with a supply of motivation and idea. Motivation and concept comprise feeling energized and pushed to reap your dreams and pursue your passions. Strong relationships can provide people with the encouragement, motivation, and sources they want to pursue their dreams and goals. This can assist people live targeted and inspired, although they're going thru worrying situations or setbacks.

Research has tested that strong relationships may have a substantial impact on highbrow health and properly-being. Studies have positioned that human beings who've sturdy social aid networks are masses less probably to increase highbrow health issues, along with despair and anxiety. Strong relationships can also assist people address strain and trauma. For example, human beings who've robust relationships after a worrying occasion, collectively with a natural catastrophe or a terrorist attack, usually generally tend to experience a good deal less intellectual misery and get higher more fast.

One of the important factor blessings of constructing sturdy relationships in Psychological Immunity is that it can assist people assemble resilience. Resilience refers to the capability to get better from difficult situations and triumph over adversity. Individuals who have sturdy relationships have a tendency to be greater resilient and better capable of deal with life's challenges. Strong relationships can provide people with a sense of protection and stability, that might help them live grounded and centered all through tough instances.

Building strong relationships also can help people broaden wholesome coping mechanisms. Coping mechanisms are the strategies that people use to control stress and emotional distress. Healthy coping mechanisms, which includes exercise, meditation, and remedy, can assist human beings control strain and decorate their highbrow fitness. Strong relationships can provide humans with the encouragement, motivation, and assets they want to increase healthy coping mechanisms.

Another vital advantage of constructing strong relationships in Psychological Immunity is that it is able to assist people triumph over stigma and discrimination. Stigma and discrimination can be massive limitations to attempting to find assist and assist for highbrow fitness issues. Strong relationships can offer people with a strong and supportive environment in which they're in a function to speak their highbrow fitness issues with out worry of judgment or discrimination. Strong relationships can also assist human beings task terrible stereotypes and attitudes approximately mental fitness.

Building strong relationships can also play a critical position in stopping highbrow fitness issues. Studies have placed that people who've strong social help networks are an entire lot less in all likelihood to expand highbrow fitness troubles, collectively with melancholy and anxiety. Strong relationships can offer individuals with the emotional and psychological belongings they need to deal with strain and exceptional annoying conditions earlier than they trade into extra excessive intellectual health issues.

Despite the numerous benefits of building sturdy relationships in Psychological Immunity , many humans struggle to collect and hold sturdy relationships. This may be because of a choice of things, which include social isolation, stigma, and discrimination. It is essential for people to take proactive steps to assemble and keep robust relationships, inclusive of joining clubs or groups, volunteering, and reaching out to pals and family.

In end, constructing sturdy relationships is a vital problem of Psychological Immunity that could assist human beings address emotional distress and intellectual harm. Strong relationships can provide people with emotional useful resource, a feel of belonging, and a deliver of motivation and concept. Building sturdy relationships also can assist people construct resilience, make bigger healthy coping mechanisms, triumph over stigma and discrimination, and prevent intellectual health problems. It is critical for humans to take proactive steps to construct and maintain sturdy relationships, as this may help them lead happier, extra healthy, and greater appealing lives.

Setting Boundaries to Protect Mental Health

Toxic relationships might also moreover have a giant impact on highbrow fitness and well-being. A toxic courting is one this is characterized with the aid of awful behaviors, along with emotional abuse, manipulation, and control. These behaviors can cause human beings to enjoy stressful, confused, and depressed, and may purpose extended-term mental damage. In this newsletter, we can find out the impact of toxic relationships on Psychological Immunity and the manner human beings can defend themselves from the terrible results of poisonous relationships.

Toxic relationships can motive people to experience various poor feelings, which include tension, strain, and depression. These horrific emotions can be because of using pretty some toxic behaviors, which encompass emotional abuse, manipulation, and control. Emotional abuse consists of the usage of terms and actions to damage, intimidate, or manage another person. Manipulation includes the usage of strategies, inclusive of guilt-tripping and gaslighting, to control a few other person's thoughts and moves. Control involves exerting electricity over every other person, which include through manner of using limiting their get right of entry to to assets or retaining apart them from buddies and circle of relatives.

Toxic relationships can also purpose people to revel in physical signs and symptoms and symptoms, at the facet of complications, fatigue, and digestive troubles. These physical signs can be resulting from the stress and anxiety that people enjoy because of toxic behaviors. Chronic pressure and anxiety also can weaken the immune device, making human beings greater susceptible to contamination and disorder.

One of the maximum first-rate influences of toxic relationships on Psychological Immunity is the development of intellectual health problems, along with despair and anxiety. Studies have determined that people who are in toxic relationships are much more likely to enjoy signs and symptoms of melancholy and anxiety than oldsters which can be in wholesome relationships. This is due to the reality toxic behaviors can cause individuals to experience hopeless, helpless, and trapped, that would reason emotions of sadness, worthlessness, and despair.

Toxic relationships also can cause human beings to boom low conceitedness and a negative self-image. This is due to the fact poisonous behaviors may be directed at an person's self confidence and self-esteem, making them revel in unworthy and unlovable. Low arrogance can result in some of intellectual health troubles, inclusive of hysteria, melancholy, and consuming problems.

Toxic relationships also can reason people to revel in trauma and placed up-demanding strain illness (PTSD). Trauma is a mental reaction to a distressing or stressful occasion, at the side of emotional abuse or physical violence. PTSD is a intellectual health condition which could develop after a worrying occasion, and is characterized with the resource of symptoms at the side of flashbacks, nightmares, and avoidance behaviors. Individuals who are in poisonous relationships are at a better threat of experiencing trauma and PTSD, that may have prolonged-time period mental outcomes.

Toxic relationships also can motive humans to engage in awful coping mechanisms, which includes substance abuse and self-damage. These coping mechanisms are frequently used as a way to numb the pain and distress due to toxic behaviors. However, they may bring about in addition psychological harm and can make it greater difficult for people to recover from the bad consequences of poisonous relationships.

In addition to the horrible influences on intellectual fitness and properly-being, poisonous relationships also can have a big effect on social and occupational functioning. Individuals who are in poisonous relationships might also additionally discover it difficult to hold healthy relationships with pals and own family, and can war to perform well at paintings or university. This can result in social isolation, monetary troubles, and a number of unique bad results.

Despite the horrible impacts of poisonous relationships, many people warfare to depart those relationships. This can be due to a range of factors, which incorporates worry, guilt, and a loss of help. It is crucial for human beings to understand the symptoms and signs of toxic relationships and to take proactive steps to protect themselves from the awful effects of toxic behaviors.

In stop, poisonous relationships might also have a exquisite effect on Psychological Immunity and may bring about some of horrible results, which include despair, tension, trauma, and espresso conceitedness. Toxic behaviors can also purpose people to have interaction in lousy coping mechanisms and can effect social and occupational functioning. It is vital for people to recognize the signs of poisonous relationships and to take proactive steps to defend themselves from the horrible effects of poisonous behaviors. This also can incorporate looking for assist from buddies and family, looking for expert help, and taking steps to move away poisonous relationships.

## Chapter 6: Developing Resilience

Defining Resilience

Resilience is the functionality to adapt and deal with adversity, trauma, and strain. It is the ability to recover from tough studies and to get higher from setbacks. Resilience is not a tough and speedy trait, but as an opportunity a tough and fast of abilities and behaviors that may be superior and bolstered over time. In this newsletter, we will explore the idea of resilience, its importance, and how humans can increase and decorate their resilience.

The Importance of Resilience

Resilience is an crucial element of highbrow fitness and well-being. It allows people to deal with strain, adversity, and trauma, and to recover from hard research. Resilience also can assist individuals to increase a greater extremely good outlook on existence, and to sense more assured and empowered.

Resilience is mainly vital in instances of disaster or trauma, collectively with natural screw ups, infection, or loss. In those situations, people who are resilient are better able to address the traumatic conditions they face, and to get higher more rapid from the revel in.

Resilience is likewise essential in ordinary existence. It can help people to deal with the pressure of labor, relationships, and high-quality demanding conditions, and to preserve a superb outlook on lifestyles. Resilience can also assist human beings to boom a revel in of cause and which means, and to enjoy extra associated with others.

Factors that Contribute to Resilience

Resilience is stimulated with the beneficial useful resource of a choice of things, which incorporates genetics, environment, and private characteristics. The following are some of the key elements that contribute to resilience:

1. Genetics: Some people may be genetically predisposed to resilience, because of variations of their DNA. However, genetics are not the great aspect that contributes to resilience, and individuals who do not have a genetic predisposition to resilience can despite the fact that increase and enhance their resilience through first-rate approach.

2. Environment: The surroundings in which humans develop up also can have an effect on their resilience. Individuals who expand up in supportive and nurturing environments, with access to sources and opportunities, may be more likely to increase resilience than those who expand up in more difficult environments.

3. Personal Characteristics: Personal inclinations, together with optimism, vanity, and a revel in of reason, also can make contributions to resilience. Individuals who've those characteristics can be better capable of address strain and adversity, and to get better more rapid from hard critiques.

four. Social Support: Social help is additionally an vital element in resilience. Individuals who've strong social networks, with supportive friends and circle of relatives participants, can be higher able to address pressure and adversity, and to get higher greater speedy from tough studies.

Developing and Enhancing Resilience

While resilience is brought about via a choice of things, it is also a difficult and fast of talents and behaviors that may be advanced and extra pleasant through the years. The following are some strategies that people can use to boom and decorate their resilience:

1. Build Strong Relationships: Building sturdy relationships with pals, family participants, and unique supportive human beings can assist to beautify resilience. These relationships can provide emotional guide, practical assistance, and a revel in of belonging and connection.

2. Practice Self-Care: Practicing self-care, which includes getting enough sleep, consuming a healthful food plan, and appealing in normal exercise, can assist to decorate resilience. These practices can assist people to control pressure, to hold a wonderful outlook on existence, and to feel extra confident and empowered.

3. Develop Coping Skills: Developing coping abilties, which incorporates trouble-solving, rest strategies, and mindfulness, can also assist to decorate resilience. These abilties can assist human beings to manipulate pressure, to cope with hard feelings, and to get better more quick from tough research.

4. Cultivate Optimism: Cultivating optimism, or a outstanding outlook on existence, also can help to decorate resilience. Optimism can help humans to keep a experience of desire and cause, even in the face of adversity, and to get better more speedy from difficult reviews.

five. Seek Support: Seeking help from mental health experts, which encompass therapists or counselors, can also assist to decorate resilience. These professionals can offer guidance, help, and assets to help people address strain, trauma, and unique annoying conditions.

In stop, resilience is an critical factor of highbrow fitness and well-being. It allows humans to address strain, adversity, and trauma, and to get over hard stories. Resilience is induced thru a variety of factors, collectively with genetics, environment, and private characteristics. However, resilience is likewise a hard and rapid of abilities and behaviors that can be superior and more advantageous through the years. By constructing sturdy relationships, schooling self-care, growing coping abilities, cultivating optimism, and seeking out manual, individuals can boom and beautify their resilience, and lead greater first rate and pleasant lives.

The Benefits of Resilience

Resilience is the ability to conform and deal with adversity, trauma, and strain. It is the capability to recover from hard evaluations and to get higher from setbacks. Resilience is not a difficult and rapid trait, however instead a difficult and rapid of abilties and behaviors that can be superior and bolstered over the years. In this article, we can find out the blessings of resilience, collectively with its impact on intellectual health, bodily health, and everyday properly-being.

## Chapter 7: The Importance Of A Strong Immune System

In current-day speedy-paced and often traumatic cutting-edge worldwide, retaining a sturdy immune system is of excessive significance for each ladies and men most of the long time of 25 and 45. A sturdy immune gadget now not handiest allows defend towards common ailments however additionally facilitates popular health and nicely-being. This subchapter explores the significance of a robust immune tool and highlights the position of superfoods in immune assist.

Your immune tool acts as a defend, defending your body in opposition to dangerous pathogens, viruses, and bacteria which can reason infection. A sturdy immune gadget is instrumental in stopping diseases collectively with the common bloodless, flu, or even extra severe conditions. It is likewise essential for restoration and healing while you do fall unwell. By that specialize in strengthening your immune machine, you can enhance your frame's natural safety mechanisms and reduce the hazard of falling prey to diverse illnesses.

Superfoods play a pivotal characteristic in supporting and enhancing the immune device. These nutrient-dense meals are complete of nutrients, minerals, antioxidants, and unique critical compounds that assist combat off infections and promote not unusual health. Incorporating superfoods into your healthy eating plan can offer the important vitamins your immune device needs to feature optimally.

Some of the most robust superfoods for immune manual encompass berries, along with blueberries and strawberries, which might be rich in antioxidants that guard in opposition to mobile harm and bolster immunity. Green leafy greens like spinach and kale are also remarkable alternatives as they're full of vitamins A, C, and E, which might be identified to enhance immune characteristic.

Additionally, incorporating materials like garlic, ginger, and turmeric can offer each anti inflammatory and immune-boosting houses. These superfoods have been used for hundreds of years for his or her restoration results on the immune gadget.

In this subchapter, we delve into the precise blessings of numerous superfoods for immune resource. We find out their nutritional profiles, highlighting the perfect nutrients, minerals, and antioxidants they include which may be critical for immune health. Moreover, we provide realistic pointers on a manner to contain those superfoods into your daily weight loss program, ensuring that you are equipping your body with the critical system to keep a sturdy immune device.

By information the significance of a strong immune system and incorporating superfoods into your weight loss plan, you may decorate your body's herbal safety mechanisms and decorate your extensive fitness and properly-being. With the statistics received from this subchapter, you will be ready to make knowledgeable choices approximately your food regimen and take proactive steps in the direction of achieving an immunity reset.

How the Immune System Works

Understanding how the immune device capabilities is crucial in current current-day worldwide, wherein our our bodies are continuously exposed to severa environmental stressors and pathogens. In this subchapter, we are capable of delve into the intricacies of the immune device, offering you with an insightful evaluation of its mechanisms and how it protects our our our bodies from harm.

The immune device is a complex community of cells, tissues, and organs that art work together to shield the body toward dangerous invaders such as micro organism, viruses, and pollution. Its primary characteristic is to apprehend and dispose of overseas substances even as retaining a touchy stability to prevent immoderate reactions that would damage our private cells.

At the center of this protection device are white blood cells, moreover referred to as leukocytes, which is probably the squaddies of our immune device. These cells are divided into classes: innate and adaptive immunity. Innate immunity acts due to the fact the first line of safety, offering rapid however non-precise responses to pathogens. On the alternative hand, adaptive immunity is a quite specialized device that develops over the years and gives a tailored reaction to specific pathogens.

Superfoods play a critical role in assisting our immune gadget. They are nutrient-dense meals which can be rich in antioxidants, vitamins, minerals, and precise bioactive compounds. Incorporating those superfoods into our diet can assist toughen our immune tool, beautify its response to pathogens, and decrease the danger of persistent illnesses.

Some of the superfoods recognized for his or her immune-supporting homes consist of berries, leafy veggies, citrus forestall cease end result, garlic, ginger, turmeric, and green tea. These food are filled with vital vitamins and antioxidants that promote the producing of white blood cells, beautify the hobby of immune cells, and defend our cells from damage because of loose radicals.

Moreover, superfoods moreover offer a myriad of various health benefits. They can help reduce contamination, support intestine fitness, beautify power tiers, and beautify everyday nicely-being. By incorporating those superfoods into your each day diet, you can't handiest supply a lift in your immune device but moreover sell first-rate fitness and strength.

In stop, facts how the immune gadget works is vital for maintaining greatest health and nicely-being inside the contemporary international. By incorporating superfoods into your diet, you may offer critical vitamins and antioxidants that guide your immune gadget's function. With a strong and well-functioning immune tool, you could better shield your frame from unstable invaders and maintain fashionable fitness and strength.

## Chapter 8: The Modern World And Immune Health

Environmental Factors and Immunity

In current day current-day international, we're continuously uncovered to numerous environmental factors that might have a big effect on our immune device. As men and women a few of the a long term of 25 and forty five, it is vital for us to recognize how those factors have an impact on our immunity and what superfoods we will embody into our diets to guide and pork up our immune machine.

One of the primary environmental factors that can have an impact on our immunity is pollutants. Whether we stay in a bustling metropolis or a suburban location, we're uncovered to air pollutants, chemical substances, and pollution on a every day foundation. These pollutants can weaken our immune gadget and make us more susceptible to infections and sicknesses. However, through eating superfoods which is probably wealthy in antioxidants, collectively with berries, leafy veggies, and turmeric, we're capable of help fight the dangerous outcomes of pollutants and boom our immune device.

Another environmental component that might impact our immunity is pressure. In cutting-edge-day rapid-paced global, stress has become a commonplace incidence for plenty folks. Chronic pressure can suppress our immune tool, making us greater vulnerable to ailments. To counteract this, we are capable of encompass superfoods like dark chocolate, avocados, and inexperienced tea in our weight loss plan, which may be seemed for his or her pressure-decreasing homes. These foods no longer simplest provide vital nutrients however moreover help sell a experience of calmness and nicely-being.

Furthermore, our immune machine may be tormented by the best of the food we eat. Processed meals, sugary snacks, and speedy meals are not unusual culprits that might weaken our immune device. To counteract this, we are capable of reputation on incorporating superfoods which might be nutrient-dense and guide immune feature. Foods like garlic, ginger, mushrooms, and citrus culmination are notable alternatives as they may be filled with crucial nutrients, minerals, and antioxidants that can decorate our frame's protection mechanisms.

Additionally, our immune system can be encouraged via our manner of life alternatives, consisting of lack of sleep and physical inaction. Incorporating superfoods like nuts, seeds, and entire grains can provide us with the essential vitamins to useful resource appropriate sleep patterns and decorate our power levels for physical interest, every of which may be crucial for keeping a strong immune tool.

In conclusion, as humans inside the age group of 25 to forty five, we need to be aware about the environmental factors that might impact our immunity. By incorporating superfoods rich in antioxidants, pressure-decreasing homes, and vital vitamins into our diets, we are able to decorate our immune machine and shield ourselves from the worrying situations posed with the useful resource of the cutting-edge global. It is critical to prioritize our fitness and well-being through making conscious alternatives that help our immune device within the face of environmental factors.

Stress and Immune Function

In extraordinarily-modern-day fast-paced and demanding international, stress has come to be an inevitable a part of our lives. From work pressures to non-public duties, pressure may have an effect on us all. But did you recognize that pressure also can have a profound effect on our immune device? In this subchapter, we will discover the hard dating among pressure and immune function, and the way incorporating superfoods into your weight loss plan can assist resource your immune machine in some unspecified time in the destiny of stressful instances.

When we revel in stress, whether or not or no longer it is acute or persistent, our frame releases stress hormones which includes cortisol. While cortisol is critical for coping with short-term pressure, prolonged publicity to excessive levels of cortisol can suppress our immune machine. This makes us greater at risk of infections, viruses, and special ailments. Moreover, stress also can impair the body's capacity to get over illnesses, most crucial to prolonged recovery instances.

Fortunately, nature has furnished us with an array of superfoods that can assist assist and boom our immune machine. These superfoods are wealthy in critical vitamins, minerals, and antioxidants that art work together to reinforce our body's protection mechanisms. Incorporating those superfoods into our every day diet regime can appreciably enhance our immune characteristic and assist us fight the bad results of stress.

One such superfood is turmeric, regarded for its strong anti-inflammatory homes. Curcumin, the energetic compound in turmeric, has been scientifically tested to decorate immune response and decrease inflammation. Another immune-boosting superfood is garlic, which includes allicin, a compound that has antimicrobial and antiviral houses. Consuming garlic often can help maintain off infections and enhance your immune gadget.

Additionally, incorporating healthy dietweight-reduction plan C-wealthy superfoods like oranges, strawberries, and kiwis can offer a much-wanted boom for your immune device. Vitamin C is a powerful antioxidant that enables defend our cells from harm attributable to stress and boosts the producing of white blood cells, which can be important for stopping off infections.

In stop, stress will have a extensive effect on our immune machine, making us more prone to illnesses. However, via incorporating immune-supporting superfoods into our each day healthy eating plan, we are able to provide a boost to our body's protection mechanisms and shield ourselves from the bad effects of stress. From turmeric to garlic and food plan C-wealthy end stop end result, nature has provided us with an abundance of superfoods which could help us reset our immune machine and thrive within the cutting-edge global.

## Chapter 9: Super Foods

What Are Superfoods?

In the fast-paced cutting-edge international, it's far turning into increasingly more critical to prioritize our fitness and well-being. One way to benefit that is through incorporating superfoods into our food regimen. But what precisely are superfoods? Let's delve into this fascinating challenge rely and discover how they may be able to help improve our immune machine.

Superfoods are nutrient-dense components that provide a plethora of health advantages. Packed with nutrients, minerals, antioxidants, and phytochemicals, they have got the power to beautify our immune tool and guard us from numerous diseases. These extraordinary elements are natural powerhouses that could have a profound effect on our common properly-being.

When it involves assisting our immune gadget, superfoods play a critical characteristic. They are in particular beneficial for individuals most of the some time of 25 and 45, as that could be a important time while our our bodies want extra manual to combat every day stressors and keep maximum reliable health. Superfoods can assist make stronger our immune device, making us an awful lot less liable to ailments and infections.

Some famous superfoods for immune guide consist of:

1. Berries: Blueberries, strawberries, and raspberries are rich in antioxidants, which help defend our cells from harm due to unfastened radicals. They moreover consist of excessive tiers of weight-reduction plan C, that is important for a sturdy immune response.

2. Leafy Greens: Spinach, kale, and Swiss chard are superb sources of vitamins A, C, and E. These vitamins are essential for supporting our immune gadget and selling wholesome cell characteristic.

three. Citrus Fruits: Oranges, lemons, and grapefruits are filled with nutrients C, known for its immune-boosting homes. Including those culmination in our every day food regimen can help decorate our immune machine.

four. Garlic: This smelly bulb is thought for its antimicrobial and antiviral houses. It can assist preserve off commonplace colds and distinct respiration infections, making it an crucial superfood for immune manual.

5. Turmeric: With its effective anti-inflammatory homes, turmeric can assist lessen irritation in the frame, boosting our immune response. It consists of a compound known as curcumin, which has been proven to have immune-boosting consequences.

Incorporating those superfoods into our healthy eating plan may want to have a great impact on our immune system and normal fitness. They can provide us with the important nutrients to reinforce our body's defense mechanisms and keep us feeling colorful and energetic.

By making conscious choices to consist of the ones superfoods in our each day food, we are able to take a proactive technique closer to our immune fitness. In the fast-paced worldwide we stay in, it is essential to prioritize our well-being and arm ourselves with the device important to thrive. Superfoods are a effective ally in this journey, supporting us increase our immune device and stay our extremely good lives.

The Role of Superfoods in Boosting Immunity

In contemporary-day speedy-paced modern-day international, it has become increasingly essential to prioritize our health and properly-being. One important factor of preserving a sturdy and resilient frame is ensuring a sturdy immune gadget. The immune system acts as our body's safety mechanism toward harmful pathogens, viruses, and illnesses. To guide and enhance this vital gadget, incorporating superfoods into our eating regimen can play a massive function.

Superfoods are nutrient-dense, herbal meals which may be filled with vital nutrients, minerals, antioxidants, and phytochemicals. They own incredible houses that would bolster our immune system, guard in competition to illnesses, and promote ordinary fitness.

One such superfood is the strong blueberry. Bursting with antioxidants, nutrients A and C, and anthocyanins, blueberries are a powerful best buddy in enhancing immune feature. Their anti-inflammatory homes assist fight oxidative stress and reduce the threat of chronic illnesses. Including a handful of these high-quality berries on your each day weight loss plan can provide a enormous decorate in your immune device.

Another immune-boosting superfood is the colourful and versatile spinach. Rich in iron, vitamins A, C, and E, and beta-carotene, spinach lets in beef up the immune tool through promoting the manufacturing of infection-stopping white blood cells. Its immoderate folate content material moreover performs a important role in DNA synthesis and repair. Incorporating spinach into your food, whether or now not in salads, smoothies, or sautés, can considerably make a contribution to a more fit immune tool.

Turmeric, the golden spice regularly determined in curries, is every other excellent superfood famend for its immune-boosting houses. Curcumin, the energetic compound in turmeric, possesses effective anti-inflammatory and antioxidant results. It enables enhance the immune response, fights off infections, and lets in the frame in restoration itself. Adding this colorful spice to your dishes no longer best enhances their taste but moreover provides precious immune assist.

In addition to blueberries, spinach, and turmeric, there can be an array of various superfoods which could bolster your immune machine. These include garlic, ginger, inexperienced tea, almonds, and kale, to call only some. Incorporating an entire lot of these superfoods into your every day food will offer your frame with a wide variety of crucial vitamins, vitamins, and minerals vital for top-nice immune function.

As human beings between the a long term of 25 and 45, it's miles essential to prioritize our fitness and properly-being. By records the function of superfoods in boosting immunity, we're able to make informed picks approximately our food regimen and manner of life. By incorporating the ones superfoods into our each day routine, we're able to manual our immune system, guard towards ailments, and revel in a extra in form and extra colorful lifestyles.

## Chapter 10: Essential Nutrients

Vitamin C: The Immune-Boosting Powerhouse

In the quick-paced international we stay in in recent times, preserving a robust immune system is essential for each ladies and men among the a while of 25 and forty five. The constant publicity to stress, pollutants, and dangerous behavior can take a toll on our health and make us more vulnerable to illnesses. That's why incorporating superfoods into our each day healthy eating plan is important, and Vitamin C stands out as one of the only immune-boosting superheroes.

Vitamin C, moreover known as ascorbic acid, is a water-soluble food regimen that plays a essential characteristic in assisting our immune gadget. It is a robust antioxidant that allows shield our cells against risky loose radicals, decreasing the hazard of persistent ailments. What makes Vitamin C clearly incredible is its ability to decorate the manufacturing of white blood cells, that are our body's frontline safety within the course of infections and illnesses.

Including substances wealthy in Vitamin C to your weight loss plan can provide severa fitness advantages. Citrus culmination like oranges, lemons, and grapefruits are well-known for his or her excessive Vitamin C content cloth. Not simplest do they taste clean, but further they provide a herbal beautify to your immune device. Other stop end result like strawberries, kiwis, and pineapples also are remarkable assets of this crucial diet.

But Vitamin C isn't restricted to clearly culmination. Vegetables which embody bell peppers, broccoli, and kale are packed with this immune-boosting nutrient. Adding the ones vegetables in your each day food no longer handiest gives a burst of flavor but moreover ensures you're fueling your frame with the critical nutrients to live healthful.

For people who find it difficult to eat sufficient amounts of Vitamin C via their diet regime, supplements may be a convenient alternative. High-terrific Vitamin C dietary supplements are quite virtually available within the market, imparting an clean and powerful way to satisfy your every day necessities.

In forestall, Vitamin C is a real immune-boosting powerhouse that everyone among the a long time of 25 and 45 have to include into their weight loss program. By together with Vitamin C-wealthy superfoods together with citrus give up quit result and veggies, you may red meat up your immune device and guard your body closer to ailments and infections. Remember, a healthful immune device is the key to thriving in the modern-day international and preserving high-quality fitness.

Zinc: A Key Mineral for Immune Function

In our speedy-paced cutting-edge-day worldwide, retaining a sturdy immune device is important for every males and females among the a long time of 25 and forty five.

The consistent exposure to stress, pollution, and processed substances makes it difficult for our our bodies to fight off infections and stay wholesome. That's wherein superfoods are to be had, and one mineral that stands out for its immune-boosting homes is zinc.

Zinc is a critical nutrient that plays a crucial feature in immune function. It acts as a catalyst for over three hundred enzymes involved in numerous bodily methods, which incorporates mobile division, growth, and repair. When it involves immunity, zinc is crucial for the manufacturing and feature of white blood cells, which can be answerable for preventing off unstable pathogens.

Research has showed that zinc supplementation can decorate the hobby of herbal killer cells, a type of white blood mobile that dreams and destroys inflamed cells. It moreover enables within the manufacturing of antibodies, which might be proteins that understand and neutralize particular pathogens. By ensuring suitable sufficient zinc intake, you may deliver your immune device an extra enhance and decrease the likelihood of falling ill.

Fortunately, incorporating zinc-wealthy superfoods into your diet plan is enormously easy. Oysters are one of the excellent assets of this mineral, containing up to 10 times extra zinc than every different meals. If you are not keen on seafood, you may flip to plant-based totally alternatives which include pumpkin seeds, spinach, chickpeas, or lentils. These food not great offer zinc but additionally offer numerous specific crucial vitamins that help common fitness.

However, it's far crucial to be conscious that on the equal time as zinc is crucial for immune characteristic, extra isn't always continuously higher. The recommended each day consumption for adults is spherical 11 mg for guys and eight mg for ladies. Excessive zinc supplementation can disrupt the balance of different minerals within the body and result in negative results, at the aspect of nausea and copper deficiency. Therefore, it's extraordinary to build up zinc from natural meals property and speak over with a healthcare professional in advance than thinking about supplementation.

In give up, zinc is a key mineral for immune characteristic, making it an important component of any superfood-centered eating regimen for males and females among the a long time of 25 and 45. By incorporating zinc-wealthy meals into your every day food, you may offer your body with the critical equipment to fight off infections and stay healthful within the cutting-edge global. Remember, stability is excessive, so motive for the endorsed each day consumption and trying to find recommendation from a healthcare professional for customized advice.

Vitamin D: The Sunshine Vitamin for Immunity

In the quest for a sturdy and resilient immune device, one regularly disregarded however essential nutrient is Vitamin D. Commonly called the "sunshine weight loss program," Vitamin D performs a vital characteristic in helping our immune device and favored health. As ladies and men a number of the a long term of 25 and forty five navigate the current-day global, it's miles important to understand the importance of this superfood for immune help.

Vitamin D is unique because of the reality our our our bodies have the extremely good capacity to offer it even as uncovered to daylight. However, because of our demanding existence and limited sun publicity, plenty folks are bad in this critical nutrient. This deficiency can drastically impact our immune device and go away us susceptible to various illnesses and infections.

Research has tested that Vitamin D performs a pivotal feature in strengthening our immune reaction. It permits alter the producing and interest of immune cells, making sure our frame can efficaciously fight off dangerous pathogens. In addition, Vitamin D has been connected to decreasing the hazard of continual sicknesses which embody cardiovascular situations, extremely good cancers, and autoimmune disorders.

Ensuring an adequate consumption of Vitamin D can be finished through a mixture of daytime exposure, weight loss program, and supplementation. While sunlight hours stays the excellent natural supply of Vitamin D, it's miles essential to strike a stability among strong solar publicity and protective our pores and pores and pores and skin from harmful UV rays. Incorporating substances rich in Vitamin D into our weight loss program is every one-of-a-kind superb manner to enhance our levels. Fatty fish like salmon, dairy merchandise, fortified cereals, and egg yolks are all high-quality resources of this superfood.

Supplementation additionally can be critical, especially for those residing in regions with restricted daytime or for people with particular fitness conditions. Consulting with a healthcare professional to determine the proper dosage and shape of Vitamin D supplementation is suggested.

As we strive to live healthful and active lives, it's miles important to prioritize the placement of Vitamin D in our immune manual routine. By maintaining top-quality stages of this sunshine vitamin, we're capable of beautify our body's defense tool, sell common nicely-being, and shield ourselves from the traumatic conditions of the present day-day worldwide.

Remember, Vitamin D isn't always handiest a nutrition; it's miles a superfood for immunity. Embrace the strength of the sunshine nutrients and liberate the whole ability of your immune device nowadays.

Omega-three Fatty Acids: Anti-Inflammatory Support

In the current international, wherein stress, pollution, and dangerous diets are rampant, preserving a strong immune tool has turn out to be greater vital than ever. Fortunately, nature has supplied us with powerful superfoods that may help decorate our immune function and promote standard properly-being. One such employer of superfoods is wealthy in omega-three fatty acids, which have received massive interest for their anti inflammatory homes.

Omega-3 fatty acids are a form of polyunsaturated fat which may be vital for our frame's superior functioning. While our frame cannot produce these fatty acids on its very own, they can be acquired from numerous meals resources, along with fatty fish like salmon, mackerel, and sardines, further to flaxseeds, chia seeds, and walnuts.

One of the critical issue advantages of omega-three fatty acids is their ability to useful aid our immune machine with the resource of decreasing infection. Chronic infection has been associated with several health issues, which includes autoimmune ailments, coronary heart sickness, or maybe fine forms of most cancers. By incorporating omega-3-rich food into your food plan, you may assist combat irritation and help your body's natural protection mechanisms.

Research has proven that omega-3 fatty acids, especially eicosapentaenoic acid (EPA) and docosahexaenoic acid (DHA), can assist alter the manufacturing of inflammatory molecules inside the body. These fatty acids play a essential role in modulating the immune reaction, assisting to preserve it balanced and save you excessive infection.

Furthermore, omega-3 fatty acids were determined to beautify the interest of immune cells, which encompass herbal killer cells and macrophages, which is probably responsible for figuring out and getting rid of risky pathogens. By strengthening those immune cells, omega-three fatty acids can assist in preventing off infections and promoting popular immune resilience.

In addition to their anti-inflammatory results, omega-three fatty acids have also been related to stepped forward cardiovascular fitness, thoughts feature, and joint health. Incorporating those superfoods into your every day weight loss program cannot handiest help your immune tool however additionally offer a number of splendid advantages to your not unusual nicely-being.

To gather the advantages of omega-three fatty acids, aim to eat fatty fish as a minimum two times every week. If you comply with a plant-based totally totally food plan, bear in mind incorporating plant property of omega-3s, in conjunction with flaxseeds, chia seeds, and walnuts, into your meals. Additionally, omega-three nutritional supplements are to be had for folks that can also additionally conflict to satisfy their nutritional necessities.

By incorporating omega-3 fatty acids into your diet regime, you could provide your body with the critical equipment to fight infection and help your immune device. These superfoods are a herbal and powerful way to beef up your frame's defenses inside the contemporary worldwide and promote top-quality fitness and properly-being for both men and women amongst 25 and forty five years vintage.

Probiotics: Gut Health and Immunity

In our fast-paced contemporary-day international, maintaining a sturdy immune gadget is essential for average fitness and well-being. As males and females between the some time of 25 and 45, we frequently locate ourselves juggling multiple obligations, which can take a toll on our immune machine. That's wherein the energy of superfoods is available in, and one superfood specifically stands proud - probiotics.

Probiotics are useful micro organism that stay in our gut and play a crucial characteristic in assisting our immune tool. They assist preserve a wholesome balance of gut micro organism, it's important for proper digestion, nutrient absorption, and essential gut health.

When our intestine is in maximum suitable situation, our immune gadget will become stronger and further resilient.

A wholesome intestine is the muse of a strong immune device. Probiotics assist decorate the production of antibodies and immune cells, which act as our body's protection tool in the direction of dangerous pathogens. By selling a healthful gut microbiome, probiotics can reduce the hazard of infections, allergies, and autoimmune troubles.

Furthermore, probiotics have been proven to enhance digestion and alleviate common intestine problems together with bloating, gasoline, and constipation. This is in particular important for men and women of their high years, as digestive ache can keep away from productiveness and high-quality of life. By incorporating probiotics into our food regimen, we can experience improved intestine fitness and better regular nicely-being.

There are diverse assets of probiotics, such as fermented substances like yogurt, kefir, sauerkraut, and kimchi. However, for people who conflict to embody these meals in their each day weight-reduction plan, probiotic dietary nutritional supplements are an first-rate opportunity. These nutritional dietary supplements offer a concentrated dose of beneficial bacteria, making sure we get keep of the top-rated quantity for immune assist.

When choosing a probiotic complement, it is crucial to search for a super product that consists of a diverse sort of lines. Different traces of micro organism have various benefits, so a numerous mixture guarantees we get hold of most immune manual. Additionally, it's miles vital to choose out a good emblem that guarantees the efficiency and viability of the probiotics until the expiration date.

# Chapter 11: Super Foods For Immune Support

Berries: Antioxidant-Rich Immune Boosters

In cutting-edge rapid-paced, contemporary-day worldwide, maintaining a sturdy immune machine is important for each males and females maximum of the a while of 25 and 45. One of nature's fine allies in this project is the common-or-lawn however extremely good berry. Bursting with flavor, those tiny end result % a punch with regards to immune assist, thanks to their immoderate antioxidant content material material.

Antioxidants are vital compounds that defend our bodies from harmful loose radicals, that can harm cells and weaken the immune tool. Berries, such as blueberries, strawberries, raspberries, and blackberries, are wealthy in those powerful antioxidants, making them superfoods for immune assist.

Blueberries, often referred to as "thoughts berries," are acknowledged for their high-quality cognitive benefits. However, their immune-boosting houses are equally terrific. Packed with vitamins C, that is famous for its functionality to enhance the immune tool, blueberries additionally include anthocyanins, a kind of antioxidant that allows fight infection and facilitates popular immune feature.

Strawberries, with their colourful crimson hue, are not most effective a adorable addition to any meal but also are a amazing source of food regimen C and other essential vitamins. Vitamin C plays a important function in enhancing the manufacturing of white blood cells, which may be answerable for preventing off infections. Including strawberries for your diet plan can deliver your immune system the enhance it needs to fight severa illnesses.

Raspberries, recounted for their tangy and barely sweet flavor, are loaded with antioxidants like diet C and quercetin. These antioxidants work together to boost the immune system and decrease infection in the body. Additionally, raspberries are rich in fiber, which permits wholesome digestion and common gut fitness, similarly helping the immune device.

Blackberries, with their deep pink colour, are complete of vitamins A and C, as well as antioxidants like anthocyanins and ellagic acid. These antioxidants assist neutralize free radicals, shield in competition to cellular damage, and lift immune function. Blackberries are also a first rate supply of dietary fiber and can make contributions to a healthy intestine, which performs a important role in the ordinary energy of the immune system.

Incorporating some of berries into your each day food plan can provide your body with a sturdy dose of antioxidants, supporting your immune tool and modern well-being. Whether enjoyed as a snack, introduced to smoothies, or used as a topping for yogurt or oatmeal, the ones antioxidant-rich end give up end result are a delicious and accessible manner to offer your immune device the useful resource it goals inside the present day-day worldwide.

Leafy Greens: Nutrient-Dense Immune Supporters

In extremely-modern-day fast-paced and disturbing global, preserving a robust immune device is vital for normal well-being. As our bodies face everyday exposure to environmental pollution, stress, and awful way of life alternatives, it turns into crucial to offer them with the vital vitamins to assist our immune defenses. One of the extremely good methods to acquire that is with the aid of manner of incorporating leafy veggies into our diets – nature's present to supercharge our immune gadget.

Leafy veggies, consisting of spinach, kale, arugula, and Swiss chard, are powerhouse greens that offer an abundance of vital vitamins, minerals, and antioxidants. These nutrient-dense vegetables play a pivotal position in selling a robust immune response, presenting a large type of benefits for women and men among the a while of 25 and forty five.

Firstly, leafy greens are rich in nutrients A, C, and E, which may be vital for retaining a healthful immune system. Vitamin A enables modify the immune machine's response to infections, while eating regimen C enables the manufacturing of white blood cells, our frame's natural protection in opposition to pathogens. Additionally, vitamins E acts as a effective antioxidant, protective our cells from oxidative damage due to free radicals.

Furthermore, leafy greens are an first-rate deliver of folate, a B-nutrition regarded to manual the producing of recent cells and DNA repair, important for a wholesome immune gadget. They additionally incorporate minerals like iron and zinc, which can be important for the right functioning of immune cells, supporting in the prevention and treatment of infections.

But the benefits do not stop there. Leafy greens are also complete of fiber, which enables a healthy gut microbiome. A well-balanced gut plants plays a crucial feature in retaining a robust immune device, because it allows modify inflammation and promotes the absorption of essential nutrients.

Incorporating leafy vegetables into your diet regime is straightforward. You can revel in them in salads, smoothies, soups, or as a aspect dish. Experiment with superb recipes and combinations to find out your favorites. To maximize their dietary rate, select herbal types every time feasible and keep in mind to clean them thoroughly in advance than intake.

In give up, leafy greens are not simplest delicious however furthermore a effective best friend in assisting a strong immune tool. By incorporating those nutrient-dense vegetables into your every day habitual, you may give a boost to your body's defenses and decorate fashionable nicely-being. So, whether or now not you're a person within the hustle and bustle of current existence, make leafy vegetables a staple on your weight-reduction plan and enjoy the transformative strength of those superfoods for immune help.

Garlic: Nature's Antibiotic for Immunity

In this modern global, wherein strain, pollution, and bad life have emerge as the norm, it has end up increasingly more critical to prioritize our immune health. Our immune device is our frame's natural protection mechanism in the direction of unstable pathogens and sicknesses, and maintaining its energy is vital. Fortunately, nature has furnished us with numerous superfoods that could improve our immunity, and one of the maximum effective amongst them is garlic.

Garlic, said for its stinky aroma and fantastic flavor, has been used for hundreds of years for its medicinal properties. This humble bulb is complete of essential nutrients and compounds that would extensively beautify our immune tool and push back infections. Garlic is wealthy in allicin, a strong compound that has been hooked up to personal antibacterial, antiviral, and antifungal homes. It acts as a herbal antibiotic, focused on dangerous pathogens and stimulating the producing of white blood cells, critical for preventing off infections.

Studies have validated that regular intake of garlic can reduce the severity and duration of not unusual illnesses which includes the not unusual bloodless and flu. Its immune-boosting houses can also help defend in opposition to greater important conditions like cardiovascular sickness, maximum cancers, and even age-associated cognitive decline. Garlic's capability to decrease blood pressure and cholesterol levels in addition contributes to its common fitness benefits.

Incorporating garlic into your every day diet regime is easy. You can upload it to your preferred dishes, whether or not or not it's far roasted, sautéed, or uncooked. For most fitness benefits, it's far endorsed to weigh down or chop garlic in advance than ingesting it, as it turns on the allicin compound. Additionally, you may take garlic supplements, that are considerably to be had in severa bureaucracy, alongside aspect capsules, powders, and oils.

However, it is critical to word that at the same time as garlic is a herbal superfood, it is not an opportunity to a wholesome life-style. Regular exercise, adequate sleep, pressure manipulate, and a balanced diet regime packed with different immune-boosting substances are further crucial for max beneficial immune characteristic.

In end, garlic is a actual superfood for immune assist. Its powerful antibacterial, antiviral, and antifungal residences make it nature's antibiotic. By incorporating garlic into your every day habitual, you could enhance your immune machine, guard in the direction of not unusual illnesses, and sell ordinary fitness and nicely-being. So, start such as this bendy and flavorful element on your food today and supply your immune device the enhance it deserves.

Turmeric: Anti-Inflammatory and Immune-Boosting Spice

In modern rapid-paced and worrying global, keeping a sturdy immune system is critical for basic health and well-being. One superfood that has acquired big reputation for its immune-boosting houses is turmeric. This golden spice, commonly observed in Indian cuisine, isn't always simplest a flavor-packed detail but furthermore a powerhouse of health advantages.

Turmeric owes its colorful coloration to a compound called curcumin, it's far chargeable for its anti inflammatory and antioxidant outcomes. These houses make turmeric an tremendous excellent pal in helping a healthy immune tool. By decreasing inflammation inside the frame, turmeric lets in defend towards chronic ailments, collectively with coronary heart disease, diabetes, and certain styles of maximum cancers.

One of the important aspect blessings of turmeric is its capability to modulate the immune response. It permits modify the pastime of immune cells, enhancing their capability to fight off infections and ailments. By strengthening the immune machine, turmeric can help save you common ailments together with the flu, colds, and allergic reactions, retaining you extra healthful and in addition resilient.

Moreover, turmeric's antioxidant houses neutralize dangerous free radicals that could damage cells and DNA. This oxidative strain now not only hurries up developing antique but additionally weakens the immune system. By incorporating turmeric into your every day diet regime, you can beautify your body's natural protection mechanisms and sluggish down the growing vintage method.

There are numerous procedures to comprise turmeric into your eating regimen. One of the most effective methods is to feature a teaspoon of turmeric powder on your favored smoothie or juice. You also can sprinkle it over roasted vegetables, combo it into soups, or use it as a flavorful seasoning for bird, fish, or tofu dishes. To decorate absorption, it's useful to consume turmeric with black pepper, because it will increase curcumin's bioavailability.

While together with turmeric to your food is a awesome begin, for max advantages, hold in thoughts combining it with special immune-boosting superfoods. For instance, you could create a sturdy immune-boosting elixir through combining turmeric with ginger, lemon, and honey. This concoction now not only tastes delicious however additionally gives a powerful dose of antioxidants and immune-assisting nutrients.

In end, turmeric is a high-quality superfood that offers a big quantity of health blessings, specially for immune beneficial resource. By incorporating this anti-inflammatory spice into your each day regular, you can assist your immune machine, reduce inflammation, and stay more healthy within the cutting-edge global. So, why not harness the strength of turmeric and deliver your immune tool the boom it deserves?

## Mushrooms: Immune-Modulating Superfood

In our modern-day-day international, wherein strain, pollutants, and terrible manner of existence selections are rampant, keeping a strong immune tool is essential. As we try to live greater healthy lives, it's critical to include superfoods into our diets that might provide us with the critical immune help. One such superfood that has won sizable interest in latest years is mushrooms.

Mushrooms were respected for masses of years in diverse cultures for their medicinal homes. Not best do they upload a totally precise flavor and texture to dishes, however additionally they provide a mess of health blessings, particularly in boosting the immune device. Whether you're a guy or a woman amongst 25 and forty five years vintage, mushrooms may be a effective best friend for your quest for pinnacle-great fitness.

One of the vital aspect reasons mushrooms are hailed as immune-modulating superfoods is their rich content material of beta-glucans. Beta-glucans are herbal compounds positioned in the cellular partitions of numerous mushroom species, which consist of Reishi, Shiitake, and Maitake. These compounds were tested to enhance the hobby of immune cells, improving the body's capability to combat off infections and ailments.

Additionally, mushrooms are filled with antioxidants, which play a important position in lowering oxidative stress and irritation within the body. By lowering inflammation, mushrooms can help save you persistent ailments which incorporates coronary coronary heart disease, diabetes, and sure types of maximum cancers. They also include vital vitamins and minerals like weight loss program D, selenium, and potassium, which further guide immune feature.

Furthermore, mushrooms have adaptogenic homes, because of this that they're capable of help the frame adapt to stressors greater efficiently. In our rapid-paced lives, strain can weaken the immune tool, making us more susceptible to ailments. By incorporating mushrooms into your food regimen frequently, you can deliver a lift to your immune machine and decorate your everyday resilience to pressure.

There are numerous techniques to enjoy mushrooms as part of your superfood regimen. You can sauté them with garlic and herbs for a delicious element dish, upload them to soups and stews, or possibly use them as a meat alternative in vegetarian dishes. For folks that determine on a greater accessible option, mushroom extracts and powders are available in complement form, making it smooth to encompass this immune-boosting superfood into your each day ordinary.

In give up, mushrooms are a powerful immune-modulating superfood which could manual and reinforce your immune tool. Whether you're a guy or a girl amongst 25 and forty five years vintage, incorporating mushrooms into your eating regimen can offer you with the critical immune aid to thrive in our present day-day worldwide. So, why now not encompass the energy of mushrooms and embark in your journey within the direction of an immunity reset?

## Chapter 12: Incorporating Super Foods Into Your Daily Routine

Superfood Smoothies and Juices

In current rapid-paced present day-day global, preserving a robust immune system is critical for each men and women a number of the some time of 25 and 45. Stress, pollutants, and awful dietary choices can take a toll on our immune health, leaving us vulnerable to ailments and infections. That's why incorporating superfood smoothies and juices into our every day habitual can be a sport-changer with reference to boosting our immune device and promoting everyday well-being.

Superfoods have received large reputation in latest years, and for proper reason. These nutrient-dense elements are packed with vitamins, minerals, antioxidants, and distinct important compounds that useful resource our immune system's functionality. By mixing those superfoods into delicious smoothies and juices, we are able to effortlessly benefit a centered dose of their immune-boosting houses.

One of the simplest superfoods for immune manual is spinach. This leafy inexperienced is wealthy in vitamins A, C, and E, similarly to folate and iron. By such as a handful of spinach in your morning smoothie, you can kick-start your day with a robust dose of immune-boosting vitamins. Combine it with exclusive superfoods like blueberries, which are loaded with antioxidants, and you've a delicious and nutritious beverage so one can maintain your immune tool sturdy.

Another superfood which could paintings wonders to your immune fitness is turmeric. Its lively compound, curcumin, has extraordinary anti-inflammatory and antioxidant homes. Adding a teaspoon of turmeric in your smoothies or juices can help lessen infection within the frame, aid digestion, and decorate your immune device's defenses.

Citrus give up result, which incorporates oranges and lemons, are also superb additions on your superfood smoothies and juices. These end result are filled with weight loss plan C, a effective antioxidant that enhances immune feature and lets in combat off infections. Start your day with a fresh citrus smoothie, and you will be well on your way to fortifying your immune device.

To decorate the immune-boosting houses of your superfood smoothies and juices, do not forget such as elements like ginger, inexperienced tea, and chia seeds. Ginger has anti inflammatory and antibacterial homes, making it an superb issue for immune help. Green tea is wealthy in antioxidants known as catechins, which can help enhance your immune system. Chia seeds are a incredible deliver of omega-three fatty acids and fiber, offering extra nutritional benefits to your superfood liquids.

In end, incorporating superfood smoothies and juices into your every day ordinary may be a easy however effective manner to manual your immune system. By blending nutrient-dense food like spinach, blueberries, turmeric, and citrus fruits, you may offer your frame with a focused dose of immune-boosting vitamins. Don't forget to check with extra factors like ginger, inexperienced tea, and chia seeds to enhance the dietary profile of your superfood liquids. Cheers to colourful fitness and a sturdy immune system!

Superfood Salads and Bowls

Superfood Salads and Bowls: Boosting Your Immunity with Delicious Nutrient Powerhouses

In this subchapter, we can delve into the area of superfood salads and bowls, displaying you the manner to create nutrient-packed food that no longer simplest satiate your taste buds however moreover offer your immune device with the guide it goals. Whether you are a guy or a woman among the a while of 25 and 45, those recipes will help you navigate the contemporary international with superior immunity.

In current day fast-paced manner of existence, it's miles important to nourish our our our bodies with the right vitamins to live wholesome and strong. Superfoods are nature's little powerhouses, jam-entire of nutrients, minerals, and antioxidants that art work wonders for our immune structures. Incorporating them into salads and bowls no longer handiest makes them visually attractive but furthermore ensures a diverse form of nutrients in a unmarried meal.

We will discover an entire lot of superfoods which may be regarded for his or her immune-assisting houses. From leafy vegetables like kale and spinach to berries wealthy in antioxidants and seeds complete of critical fatty acids, every element has its precise characteristic in fortifying your immune machine. We may also even offer guidelines on sourcing easy produce and natural additives to maximise the nutritional advantages of your meal.

Our recipes will inspire you to create colourful salads and bowls which can be every delicious and nutritious. From a colourful quinoa salad with roasted greens and avocado to a sparkling Asian-stimulated soba noodle bowl with edamame and seaweed, these recipes will tantalize your flavor buds whilst boosting your immunity. We may additionally even encompass hints on meal prepping and progressive element substitutions, allowing you to evolve the recipes for your personal possibilities and dietary desires.

By incorporating superfood salads and bowls into your every day normal, you may not most effective manual your immune device but additionally experience prolonged electricity ranges, progressed digestion, and extra suitable preferred nicely-being. So, be part of us in this culinary journey to discover the energy of superfoods and release the general potential of your immune device.

Remember, your fitness is your maximum precious asset, and with the right superfood salads and bowls, you may enhance your body against the challenges of the modern-day world. Together, let's nourish ourselves and construct a robust immune device for you to aid us for years yet to come.

Superfood Snacks and Energy Bars

In extraordinarily-modern-day fast-paced and annoying global, it can be hard to preserve ideal fitness and immunity. That's why incorporating superfood snacks and energy bars into your each day recurring could make a international of distinction. These nutrient-dense powerhouses aren't only scrumptious but additionally provide the vital gasoline and guide to boost your immune device. Whether you're a guy or a lady among the some time of 25 and 45, coming across the advantages of superfoods for immune useful resource is important to undertaking traditional well being.

Superfood snacks and energy bars are accessible and without issues on hand alternatives for busy people seeking to growth their immune device. Packed with vitamins, minerals, antioxidants, and other important vitamins, the ones snacks are designed to offer sustained energy whilst improving your body's herbal safety mechanisms. They are a surely ideal on-the-bypass answer for those instances while you need a short and healthful choose out-me-up.

One famous superfood snack is the goji berry, known for its immune-boosting houses. These small crimson berries are wealthy in nutrition C, this is critical for supporting a wholesome immune system. Goji berries moreover encompass antioxidants that assist fight the damaging outcomes of free radicals, decreasing the chance of continual ailments.

# Chapter 13: Lifestyle Factors For A Strong Immune System

Exercise and Immunity

In contemporary-day speedy-paced and worrying international, maintaining a robust immune device is vital for each women and men most of the a long time of 25 and forty five. The consistent publicity to environmental pollutants, processed meals, and sedentary life can weaken our body's natural protection mechanism, primary to a better risk of infections and illnesses. However, there may be a powerful super buddy that may significantly improve our immune device - workout.

Regular exercise has been established to have a profound effect on our ordinary health and well-being. Not simplest does it assist in keeping a wholesome weight and lowering the danger of chronic illnesses, but it additionally plays a crucial feature in strengthening our immune device. When we've interplay in physical interest, severa excessive excellent adjustments arise inner our frame that right now make a contribution to extra appropriate immune function.

One of the number one advantages of workout on the immune device is its functionality to decorate glide. As we training session, our coronary coronary heart charge will growth, pumping extra oxygen-rich blood to all additives of the body, which incorporates our immune organs. This progressed blood float guarantees that essential nutrients and immune cells are correctly introduced to wherein they may be wished the most, enhancing our body's capacity to fight off infections.

Exercise additionally stimulates the discharge of endorphins, which may be natural chemical materials in our brain that sell a revel in of nicely-being and decrease pressure. Chronic strain can weaken our immune system, making us more susceptible to contamination. By incorporating everyday workout into our routine, we're able to lessen stress stages, thereby improving our immune response.

Furthermore, exercise has been proven to boom the manufacturing of antibodies and white blood cells, which can be critical components of our immune system. These cells play a essential function in identifying and destroying dangerous pathogens, retaining us healthful and guarded.

To maximize the immune-boosting advantages of exercising, it's miles crucial to cognizance on a balanced and sundry exercise habitual. Incorporate a combination of cardiovascular wearing activities, energy schooling, and versatility sporting sports to make certain regular fitness and immune manual. Additionally, it's far surely beneficial to engage in mild-intensity exercise for at least a hundred fifty mins in step with week, as encouraged with the useful resource of using experts.

In give up, regular workout is a powerful device in strengthening our immune tool. By incorporating bodily interest into our each day lives, we are capable of enhance our frame's herbal protection mechanisms, reduce the threat of infections, and experience a greater healthful and greater colourful lifestyles. So, lace up your walking shoes, hit the fitness center, or be a part of a yoga elegance – your immune system will thanks!

Sleep and Immune Function

In extremely-modern fast-paced global, it is simple to miss the significance of sleep in retaining a robust immune device. However, studies has installed time and time all over again that a lack of best sleep also can have a poor impact on our body's capability to combat off infections and illnesses. In this subchapter, we are capable of discover the fascinating connection among sleep and immune feature, and the way incorporating superfoods into your food regimen can assist guide a wholesome immune tool.

When we sleep, our our our bodies flow into restore mode, working hard to heal and rejuvenate. During this time, our immune system releases proteins known as cytokines, which help promote sleep and fight off infections. Without enough sleep, our our our our bodies produce fewer cytokines, leaving us more at risk of illnesses on the facet of the commonplace bloodless and flu. Moreover, loss of sleep also can result in continual inflammation, which further weakens the immune device.

But how can superfoods assist on this case? Superfoods are nutrient-dense elements that provide an array of health blessings, which includes immune guide. By incorporating those elements into your each day diet regime, you can deliver your frame the important nutrients, minerals, and antioxidants it wants to give a boost to your immune tool. Some superfoods which might be particularly beneficial for immune feature embody:

1. Berries: Packed with antioxidants, berries inclusive of blueberries, strawberries, and raspberries can help reduce contamination and increase immune function.

2. Leafy greens: Spinach, kale, and different leafy vegetables are wealthy in nutrients A, C, and E, in addition to fiber and antioxidants, which all contribute to a wholesome immune machine.

three. Citrus end result: Oranges, lemons, and grapefruits are extraordinary resources of vitamin C, a effective antioxidant that would decorate immune feature.

four. Garlic: This smelly bulb not most effective affords taste in your dishes however moreover consists of compounds that can stimulate the immune gadget and help fight off infections.

5. Turmeric: Known for its anti-inflammatory houses, turmeric can assist a healthy immune reaction and reduce the danger of continual ailments.

In surrender, sleep is a crucial problem of maintaining a strong immune device. By prioritizing exceptional sleep and incorporating immune-supporting superfoods into your healthy eating plan, you could optimize your frame's capacity to combat off infections and sicknesses. Remember, a properly-rested body and a nourished immune system are the keys to thriving in the contemporary global.

Stress Management and Immunity

In present day day speedy-paced and demanding worldwide, strain has become an inevitable part of our daily lives. From paintings pressures to non-public duties, stress can take a toll on our physical and intellectual properly-being. But did you comprehend that strain furthermore has a big effect on our immune machine? In this subchapter, we can discover the vital dating among strain management and immunity, and the manner incorporating superfoods into your healthy dietweight-reduction plan can assist your immune gadget.

When we're confused, our our bodies release a hormone known as cortisol, also called the stress hormone. While cortisol is important for our combat-or-flight response, chronic pressure can bring about an overproduction of this hormone, which can weaken our immune gadget. Research has tested that extended stress can suppress the immune device, making us greater prone to ailments and infections.

This is where pressure control techniques come into play. Learning a way to efficiently control pressure can not best decorate our mental health but additionally beautify our immune tool. Engaging in sports activities sports which include yoga, meditation, or deep breathing physical activities can help lessen pressure levels and promote rest. Additionally, normal exercise and getting sufficient sleep are crucial in maintaining a wholesome immune tool.

## Chapter 14: Recipes For Immune Support

Immune-Boosting Smoothie Recipes

In modern fast-paced worldwide, maintaining a sturdy immune machine is essential for each ladies and men among the a long time of 25 and forty five. With the constant exposure to strain, pollutants, and threatening life-style options, it is no marvel that our immune structures once in a while need a hint greater help. Luckily, nature has furnished us with a big choice of superfoods which can assist increase our immune function and preserve us healthful and colorful.

In this subchapter, we are able to discover some delicious and nutritious smoothie recipes which can be packed with immune-boosting superfoods. These recipes are designed to provide your body with the critical vitamins it wants to assemble a sturdy safety against ailments and infections.

1. Green Goddess Smoothie:

This smooth smoothie is packed with leafy veggies like spinach and kale, which can be wealthy in nutrients A, C, and E – all regarded to beneficial aid immune function. Adding a handful of antioxidant-wealthy berries like blueberries and strawberries further enhances the immune-boosting houses of this smoothie.

2. Citrus Zinger Smoothie:

Citrus quit end result like oranges, lemons, and grapefruits are loaded with weight loss program C, a effective antioxidant that permits improve the immune device. This zesty smoothie combines the tangy flavors of citrus fruits with a hint of ginger, which has anti-inflammatory homes and aids digestion.

three. Tropical Turmeric Smoothie:

Turmeric, diagnosed for its colourful shade and effective anti inflammatory homes, is the well-known person detail on this tropical smoothie. Combined with pineapple, mango, and coconut water, this smoothie is not quality delicious however moreover affords a wholesome dose of nutrients and minerals that help immune function.

four. Berry Blast Smoothie:

Berries are a rich supply of antioxidants that assist shield the body in competition to dangerous loose radicals. This antioxidant-packed smoothie combines numerous berries like raspberries, blackberries, and strawberries with a handful of spinach for an introduced improve of vitamins and minerals.

By incorporating those immune-boosting smoothie recipes into your each day ordinary, you can offer your frame with the critical vitamins it desires to help a robust immune gadget. Remember, searching after your fitness is a lifelong journey, and those superfood-packed smoothies are simply one piece of the puzzle. Combine them with a balanced eating regimen, normal exercising, and adequate sleep to make certain superior immune function and common nicely-being.

So, take hold of your blender, stock up on the ones superfoods, and get geared up to offer your immune gadget the increase it merits! Cheers to a extra in shape, extra colourful you!

Superfood Salad Recipes

In this subchapter, we are able to find out an entire lot of delicious and nutrient-packed superfood salad recipes if you need to now not most effective tantalize your flavor buds however moreover offer super immune help. These recipes are particularly curated for men and women many of the a while of 25 and 45 who're attempting to find to boost their immunity inside the cutting-edge-day international.

1. Quinoa and Kale Power Salad:

This colourful salad combines the goodness of protein-wealthy quinoa, antioxidant-packed kale, and a medley of colourful vegetables. Topped with a zesty lemon dressing and sprinkled with pumpkin seeds, this salad is a dietary powerhouse with a purpose to go away you feeling energized.

2. Berry Avocado Spinach Salad:

Packed with superfoods like spinach, berries, and avocado, this smooth salad is a deal with for each your taste buds and your immune machine. The combination of antioxidants from the berries and wholesome fats from the avocado will offer the vital nourishment to help your immune device.

three. Roasted Sweet Potato and Chickpea Salad:

Roasted sweet potatoes and protein-wealthy chickpeas are the stars of this hearty salad. Mixed with a tangy tahini dressing and tossed with leafy veggies, this salad is a satisfying combination of flavors and textures for you to depart you feeling glad and fortified.

4. Citrus Quinoa Salad:

This citrus-infused salad competencies a aggregate of quinoa, colourful citrus culmination, and crunchy greens. Bursting with vitamins C and antioxidants, this salad is an amazing desire for bolstering your immune device closer to the stresses of the modern-day-day worldwide.

five. Superfood Detox Salad:

Loaded with detoxifying materials like kale, broccoli, and beets, this salad is a incredible desire for those looking to cleanse their our our bodies and enhance their immunity. Tossed in a zingy lemon-ginger dressing, this colorful salad will assist you revel in refreshed and revitalized.

Each of these superfood salad recipes has been carefully crafted to offer a scrumptious and nutritious way to assist your immune gadget. By incorporating the ones recipes into your everyday food plan, you could make stronger your body in opposition to the disturbing situations of the cutting-edge global. So, take maintain of your salad bowl and embark on a journey toward maximum splendid fitness and nicely-being with those immune-boosting superfood salads.

Nutrient-Dense Dinner Recipes

In cutting-edge rapid-paced present day international, preserving a robust immune gadget is vital for every males and females some of the some time of 25 and forty five. Our our our bodies want right nourishment to fight the daily stressors and environmental pollutants that may weaken our immune defenses. This subchapter, titled "Nutrient-Dense Dinner Recipes," is devoted to offering you with delicious and smooth-to-make meals which might be full of superfoods to guide your immune system.

Eating a nutrient-dense dinner is critical for replenishing your body's electricity stages and supplying it with the nutrients, minerals, and antioxidants it desires for maximum appropriate immune characteristic. These recipes are carefully curated to encompass a number of superfoods seemed for their immunity-boosting homes, ensuring you get maintain of the maximum advantages out of your meals.

One of the recipes you can find out on this subchapter is a hearty quinoa and vegetable stir-fry. Quinoa, a protein-rich grain, is mixed with an array of colourful veggies which encompass broccoli, bell peppers, and carrots. This dish offers an abundance of essential nutrients like vitamins A and C, which is probably crucial for keeping a robust immune tool.

For the ones attempting to find a extra indulgent opportunity, we have got a mouthwatering salmon with avocado salsa recipe. Salmon, filled with omega-three fatty acids, is understood for its anti inflammatory homes. Paired with a smooth avocado salsa loaded with vitamins E, this dish not simplest satisfies your flavor buds but moreover offers a effective immune-boosting punch.

We also understand that point may be a constraint for many individuals, it truly is why we have protected a quick and easy lentil soup recipe. Lentils are an awesome supply of plant-based protein and are rich in iron, zinc, and folate – all important nutrients for immune help. This comforting soup is good for those busy weeknights on the equal time as you want a nourishing meal without spending hours in the kitchen.

Whether you're a guy or a girl, prioritizing your immune health is critical in modern-day worldwide. By incorporating those nutrient-dense dinner recipes into your normal, you may offer your frame with the superfoods it needs to guide a sturdy immune device. Take fee of your fitness and take pleasure in the ones delicious food on the way to nourish every your frame and soul.

## Chapter 15: Building Immunity Inside The Long Term

Sustainable Habits for Immune Health

In contemporary fast-paced modern-day international, in which pressure, pollution, and awful food alternatives are rampant, it's miles vital to prioritize our immune health. As we age, our immune system will become greater prone, making us vulnerable to ailments and infections. However, via manner of adopting sustainable conduct and incorporating superfoods into our each day recurring, we are able to enhance our immune device and shield our not unusual nicely-being.

1. Nourish Your Body with Superfoods: Superfoods are nutrient-wealthy powerhouses that provide essential vitamins, minerals, and antioxidants that manual our immune tool. Incorporate factors like berries, leafy greens, citrus quit result, turmeric, ginger, garlic, and mushrooms into your weight loss plan. These superfoods are full of immune-boosting houses that can assist make stronger your frame's protection mechanisms.

2. Practice Regular Exercise: Engaging in normal bodily activity no longer fine blessings your bodily health but additionally strengthens your immune tool. Exercise will

increase flow into, permitting immune cells to move freely for the duration of your frame. Aim for at least 1/2-hour of mild exercise, which encompass walking, taking walks, or yoga, at the least 5 days in step with week to help your immune health.

three. Prioritize Sleep: Quality sleep is essential for keeping a robust immune tool. During sleep, our body protection and regenerates cells, consisting of immune cells. Aim for 7-8 hours of uninterrupted sleep each night to make sure your body has sufficient time to rejuvenate and make stronger its defenses.

four. Manage Stress Levels: Chronic stress can weaken our immune tool, making us extra susceptible to infections. Find healthful procedures to manipulate stress, collectively with education meditation, deep respiratory wearing activities, or wearing out hobbies you experience. Taking time for self-care and relaxation can substantially effect your immune fitness.

5. Stay Hydrated: Drinking sufficient water is important for assisting standard fitness, which incorporates immune function. Water permits flush out pollution, aids in digestion, and ensures proper flow into of nutrients in some unspecified time in the future of your body. Aim for as a minimum eight glasses of water regular with day to keep your immune device hydrated and functioning optimally.

In conclusion, adopting sustainable conduct for immune fitness is vital for males and females some of the a while of 25 and forty five. By incorporating superfoods into your eating regimen, jogging closer to normal workout, getting sufficient sleep, dealing with stress tiers, and staying hydrated, you can aid and deliver a boost on your immune tool. Prioritizing your immune fitness will now not best guard you from illnesses however additionally beautify your ordinary nicely-being within the current-day-day global. Start making those sustainable conduct a part of your each day normal, and revel in the blessings of a sturdy immune device for years to come.

Consistency and Patience in Building Immunity

In our fast-paced modern-day international, preserving a strong immune gadget has grow to be greater crucial than ever. The consistent exposure to pressure, pollutants, and bad manner of lifestyles alternatives can wreak havoc on our our our bodies, leaving us prone to ailments and infections. However, by way of incorporating superfoods into our every day recurring, we can enhance our immune device and shield ourselves from numerous fitness annoying situations.

Building immunity isn't an in a single day approach; it requires consistency and patience. Just like every extraordinary problem of our fitness, we cannot assume proper away consequences. It's a journey that requires dedication and a holistic technique. By adopting a few simple however powerful behavior, we're capable of steadily improve our immune device and enhance our regular properly-being.

First and maximum vital, it is critical to contain superfoods into our weight-reduction plan. These nutrient-dense food are complete of vitamins, minerals, and antioxidants that offer super immune guide. Superfoods like kale, spinach, berries, and turmeric can assist enhance our immune device and thrust back infections. Consistently in conjunction with the ones factors in our meals will step by step make more potent our frame's protection mechanisms.

www.ingramcontent.com/pod-product-compliance
Lightning Source LLC
Chambersburg PA
CBHW051726020426
42333CB00014B/1179